In Clinical Practice Series

Asthma and COPD

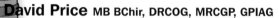

David Price MB BChir, DRCOG, MRCGP, GPIAG
General Practice Airways Group Professor of Primary Care Respiratory
Medicine, Department of General Practice and Primary Care,
University of Aberdeen, UK

Juliet Foster BA (Hons)
Primary Care Researcher of Respiratory Medicine,
Department of General Practice and Primary Care,
University of Aberdeen, UK

Jane Scullion RGN, BA (Hons), MSc
Respiratory Nurse Consultant, University Hospitals of Leicester,
Glenfield Site Institute for Lung Health, and part-time
General Practice Airways Group Clinical Research Fellow,
Department of General Practice and Primary Care,
University of Aberdeen, UK

Daryl Freeman MB ChB, DRCOG, MRCGP
General Practitioner and General Practice Airways Group Clinical
Research Fellow, Department of General Practice and Primary Care,
University of Aberdeen, UK

**CHURCHILL
LIVINGSTONE**
Edinburgh London New ... to 2004

D1334052

Churchill Livingstone
An imprint of Elsevier Limited.

 is a registered trademark of Elsevier Limited.

ISBN 0443 074682

Cataloguing in Publication Data
Catalogue records for this book are available from the US Library of Congress and the British Library.

Note
Medical knowledge is constantly changing. As new information becomes available, changes in treatment, procedures, equipment and the use of drugs become necessary. The authors and the publishers have taken care to ensure that the information given in this text is accurate and up to date. However, readers are strongly advised to confirm that the information, especially with regard to drug usage, complies with the latest legislation and standards of practice.

Front cover images reproduced from Comprehensive Respiratory Medicine, Richard Albert, Stephen Spiro and James Jett, Mosby, London, 1999, and from Respiratory Medicine, J Gibson, D Geddes, U Costabel, P Sterk, B Corrin, Saunders, London, 2003.
Figure 12 reproduced courtesy of Clement Clarke International Ltd.
Figures 13 and 16 reproduced courtesy of AstraZeneca AIR. Available from http//:www.az-air.com.
Figure 14 reproduced courtesy of Micromed.
Figure 48 reproduced courtesy of Sunrise Medical Ltd.

The publishers would like to thank Dr David Halpin for his generous permission to adapt the drug tables on pages 105–120. These were originally published in Rapid Reference COPD, copyright Mosby, 2002.

Printed in China

Acknowledgements

The authors wish to thank Miss MA Ross, Miss S Knowles and Dr Mike Thomas for their help in the preparation of this book.

Contents

Preface

Asthma and COPD are important diseases in primary care. This practical handbook is aimed at the health care practitioner and documents the common respiratory disorders of asthma and COPD in the community. Asthma and COPD are presented in distinct sections as they are clearly different disease processes with dissimilar causes and treatments.

The main objectives of this book are to help practitioners correctly identify patients with asthma and COPD, so that patients can be given optimal advice, support, education and treatment. It will be useful for GPs, practice nurses, community nurses, community pharmacists, community physiotherapists and occupational therapists.

We hope that as a result patients will ultimately:
- experience minimal symptoms with maximal improvements in their health and quality of life;
- reduce the risk of exacerbations and even death from their condition;
- be increasingly competent in managing their disease and in using their medication appropriately;
- be more satisfied with service provision;
- use health care services more appropriately.

David Price
General Practice Airways Group Professor of Primary Care Respiratory Medicine,
Department of General Practice and Primary Care,
University of Aberdeen, UK

Juliet Foster
Primary Care Researcher of Respiratory Medicine,
Department of General Practice and Primary Care,
University of Aberdeen, UK

Jane Scullion
Respiratory Nurse Consultant, University Hospitals of Leicester,
Glenfield Site Institute for Lung Health,
and part-time General Practice Airways Group Clinical Research Fellow,
Department of General Practice and Primary Care,
University of Aberdeen, UK

Daryl Freeman
General Practitioner and General Practice Airways Group Clinical Research Fellow,
Department of General Practice and Primary Care,
University of Aberdeen, UK

Biographies

David Price MB BChir, DRCOG, MRCGP, GPIAG is Professor of Primary Care Respiratory Medicine at the University of Aberdeen and a General Practitioner at Thorpewood Surgery, Norwich, UK. In 1984 Professor Price graduated in medicine from Cambridge University and trained as a GP, qualifying in 1989. Apart from a year working in paediatrics in Sydney, Australia, he has remained in general practice in Norwich. In February 2000, he was appointed General Practice Airways Group Professor of Primary Care Respiratory Medicine at the University of Aberdeen. Professor Price is extensively involved in primary care education and research and is an active member of the General Practice Airways Group and International Primary Care Respiratory Group. He also heads a consortium of seven primary care research centres in the UK. Having established a respiratory clinic 10 years ago, Professor Price's special area of interest is primary care respiratory management, particularly "real-life" effectiveness and cost-effectiveness, compliance and patient attitudes to their disease.

Juliet Foster BA (Hons) is a Primary Care Researcher of Respiratory Medicine at the University of Aberdeen, UK. After receiving a first-class degree in psychology at the University of Luton in 1999 with a dissertation on psycho-social aspects of asthma, Juliet joined the respiratory team at the University of Aberdeen. For the past two years Juliet has managed primary care research projects on international delivery of care for COPD, side-effects of inhaled corticosteroids and the management of asthma. She is now also undertaking research for her PhD at the University of Groningen in the Netherlands.

Jane Scullion RGN, BA (Hons), MSc is Respiratory Nurse Consultant at University Hospitals of Leicester Glenfield Site Institute for Lung Health, and part-time Clinical Fellow at the Department of General Practice and Primary Care, University of Aberdeen, UK. In 1981, a year as a clerical officer working with tuberculosis patients in Leicester led to nurse training, qualifying in 1986, and then posts in neurology and haematology and respiratory medicine. In 2000, Jane was appointed to the first Respiratory Nurse Consultant post in the UK, and shortly after joined the team at Foresterhill as a Clinical Fellow. Jane currently works with patients handicapped by their respiratory disease, reflecting an interest in the psychological sequelae of chronic illness.

Daryl Freeman MB ChB, DRCOG, MRCGP is a part-time General Practitioner in North Norfolk, UK and has a further part-time commitment as a General Practice Airways Group Clinical Research Fellow. In a previous post Dr Freeman set up and evaluated a large practice-based COPD service, which aimed to provide excellent care to patients and also provided information on the prevalence of COPD in the practice and the effect of managed care on various outcome measures. The project has also helped to evaluate a screening questionnaire for COPD and asthma. Dr Freeman is the lead investigator for a study looking at the decision-making process behind changes in asthma medication, and the effects of those changes.

Introduction and background

Respiratory illness is responsible for much acute and chronic illness in the UK, with more patients consulting their GP for respiratory problems than for any other disease group. In fact there are over 38 million consultations per year in general practice for respiratory problems, with over one fifth of these occurring at the patient's home.[1] Lung problems are related not just to smoking. They are connected to a wide variety of other causes ranging from genetics and the environment, to poverty and nutrition. Respiratory disease kills one in four people in the UK, a mortality rate higher than that of coronary heart disease and cancer.[1] What makes this more disturbing is that the UK death rate from respiratory disease is almost twice the European Union average (Figure 1).

"** Respiratory disease kills one in four people in the UK, a mortality rate higher than coronary heart disease and cancer **"

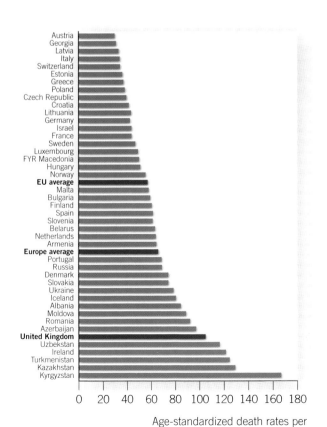

Fig. 1. Death rates from respiratory disease. Reproduced from The Burden of Lung Disease with permission from the British Thoracic Society.

Austria
Georgia
Latvia
Italy
Switzerland
Estonia
Greece
Poland
Czech Republic
Croatia
Lithuania
Germany
Israel
France
Sweden
Luxembourg
FYR Macedonia
Hungary
Norway
EU average
Malta
Bulgaria
Finland
Spain
Slovenia
Belarus
Netherlands
Armenia
Europe average
Portugal
Russia
Denmark
Slovakia
Ukraine
Iceland
Albania
Moldova
Romania
Azerbaijan
United Kingdom
Uzbekistan
Ireland
Turkmenistan
Kazakhstan
Kyrgyzstan

0   20   40   60   80   100   120   140   160   180

Age-standardized death rates per 100,000 population (1996)

Asthma is a common and chronic inflammatory condition affecting the airways. More than 3 million people in the UK, 10% of children and 5% of adults, are currently diagnosed as having asthma,[2] with considerable increases in prevalence over the last 20 years.[3] Asthma is still substantially underdiagnosed, although recently there have been some marked improvements.[4]

> *In the UK 10% of children and 5% of adults are diagnosed as having asthma*

Chronic obstructive pulmonary disease (COPD) is characterized by inflammation, bronchoconstriction, airflow obstruction and structural changes in the airways. The most important risk factor for COPD is cigarette smoking. COPD is increasingly common because of the growing prevalence of smoking and the progressively ageing population. By 2020, COPD is expected to be responsible for 7% of all deaths and become the third-leading cause of world mortality.[5] Recent research suggests that 50% of all elderly smokers may develop COPD.[6] Underdiagnosis and misdiagnosis are common; many patients, including those with severe disease, have an erroneous asthma diagnosis or no diagnosis at all.[7] Underdiagnosis is of particular concern because the slow progressive nature of COPD means it can remain undetected for years.[8,9] Smoking cessation is the most effective intervention against development and speed of COPD progression. Undiagnosed patients are unlikely to receive optimal support for smoking cessation at an early stage in their disease, with worse long-term outcomes.

> *Many COPD patients have an erroneous asthma diagnosis, or no diagnosis at all*

Patients with asthma or COPD often require frequent contact with primary and secondary care services, although most can be managed in primary care.[10,11] Good organization of care is vital to ensure seamless, consistent, high-quality delivery. Guidelines acknowledge the effectiveness of shared care for patients with more severe asthma,[12] and changes in primary care have created opportunities for developing improved models for asthma and COPD care.

ASTHMA

Definition

The term "asthma" has been recognized since ancient times, being derived from the Greek word "ασθμα" meaning short-drawn breath or panting.[13] The word has been in use since the time of Hippocrates (460–370 BC) but it probably encompassed many different causes of breathlessness during this period.

Asthma is predominantly an inflammatory disease of the airways. The 2003 British Thoracic Society and Scottish Intercollegiate Guidelines Network asthma management guidelines[14] use the international consensus definition to describe asthma as:

"a chronic inflammatory disorder of the airways. In susceptible individuals inflammatory symptoms are usually associated with widespread but variable airflow obstruction and an increase in airway response to a variety of stimuli. Obstruction is often reversible either spontaneously or with treatment."[15]

The inflammatory nature of asthma has been known for some time, with biopsy studies, published as early as 1912, revealing loss of the epithelial layer, epithelium swelling, plasma exudation and eosinophilia.[16]

A major challenge in defining, diagnosing and managing asthma is that it is not a static, uniform disease. Rather it is a dynamic, heterogeneous clinical syndrome with several clinical presentations that may vary between patients and within individuals at any point in time.[13] Patients with well-controlled asthma may be apparently asymptomatic with normal lung function between exacerbations, which are triggered by a range of factors including exercise, allergens and viral infections.

> **Patients with well-controlled asthma may be apparently asymptomatic between exacerbations**

Epidemiology and natural history

Recent estimates suggest that 10% of children worldwide have asthma.[17] Studies clearly indicate an increase in prevalence over the past 20–30 years.[18] This trend appears to result from a true increase in prevalence and also a recent tendency to label more episodes of wheezing as asthma.[19] This figure should be interpreted in relation to geographical location because prevalence rates are higher in children living in developed countries than in those living in developing and non-English-speaking countries.

Prevalence is also higher in certain countries despite similar living conditions[20,21] – for example, Australia and New Zealand compared with the United States and Canada. Such global variation indicates that environmental factors are involved in the development of asthma, although the variables responsible are not clearly defined.

Although around 10% of older children are diagnosed as having asthma, the proportion falls to around 5% in adults. This suggests asthma may not be a lifetime condition for all patients; around 25–30% of childhood asthma is thought to persist into adulthood.[22–24] Several factors appear to be linked with the persistence of symptoms, including coexisting atopic disease, age at first presentation (most children aged 2 years or younger with wheeze become asymptomatic later in childhood) and frequency and severity of episodes.[25]

> **The global variation in prevalence of asthma indicates that environmental factors are involved in development**

Over the last 30 years, epidemiological research has consistently reported a worldwide increase in asthma. Moreover, the few studies measuring prevalence change in adult asthma indicate it has increased more than two-fold in 20 years.[26–29]

Reasons proposed for this increase include proliferation of house dust mites and outdoor and indoor pollutants (for example, maternal cigarette smoking), childhood atopy, changes in diet, reduced infection exposure and increasingly sterile environments.[30, 31]

Although prevalence has increased, there was a small reduction in deaths from asthma in people under age 75 between 1988 and 1995. Nonetheless, mortality has been slow to fall and remains substantially higher in the UK than in virtually all its European neighbour countries.[1] In tandem, there appears to have been a small reduction in the rate of exacerbations presenting in primary care.[32]

It is possible that these reductions are related to increased awareness and use of prophylactic medications, because prescriptions for anti-inflammatory drugs as a proportion of all asthma drugs have increased simultaneously.[33] It is troubling, however, that the UK lags behind much of Europe in improving asthma outcomes.

> *Asthma mortality remains substantially higher in the UK than in virtually all our European neighbour countries*

Aetiology

Asthma is a heterogeneous, multifactorial disease characterized by a vast array of manifestations or phenotypes. Key components of its development include genetic factors, which are predominantly atopy and a parental history of asthma, and environmental factors including allergen exposure.

Larsen defined atopy as:

"the production of abnormal amounts of IgE antibodies in response to contact with environmental allergens, demonstrated by increased total or specific serum IgE and a positive skin-prick test to one of a battery of standardized allergens".

Evidence suggests at least half of all asthma cases are linked to atopy.[34]

> *Asthma is a heterogeneous, multifactorial disease characterized by a vast array of manifestations or phenotypes*

Environmental and genetic factors

Demographic factors such as low income, age, race and socioeconomic status[35–38] are associated with the development of asthma. Nevertheless, the increasing prevalence of the disease over the last 20 years suggests that aeroallergens,[39] indoor and outdoor air pollution,[40,41] viruses,[42] substances used in the workplace[43] (domestic[44,45] and occupational[46,47]) and exposure to endotoxin (a component of the membrane of Gram-negative bacteria) may play a role in the aetiology and pathogenesis of asthma.

Susceptibility to asthma may be determined early in life. Exposure to indoor allergens,[48, 49] passive smoking, and especially maternal smoking,[50] are associated with asthma development. Results of studies conducted in twins suggest the specific environment experienced by the individual is important, and that avoiding allergens and cigarette smoke may decrease the risk of childhood asthma.[51,52]

Although environmental factors are important, both twin and family studies indicate a strong genetic component. Community-based studies of twins estimate the heritability of asthma to be between 35% and 75%.[53] To date, studies have identified more than a dozen genomic regions linked to asthma.[54]

This genetic component may be due to an additive gene effect (combinations of genes may be needed to produce a person at risk of developing asthma), although it is not known which genes lead to asthma susceptibility.[55]

Gene–environment interactions

Genetic factors strongly influence asthma response, but their effect largely depends on environmental interaction (Figure 2).

The *hygiene hypothesis,* which postulates an inverse relationship between incidence of infectious diseases in early life and subsequent development of allergies and asthma, may provide part of the explanation for an increase in atopy and asthma in westernized countries.[56] An inadequate exposure to immune stimulants in early life may lead to a

Fig. 2. Factors affecting the asthmatic response.

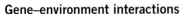

Genetic factors	Environmental factors
• Atopy	• House dust mites • Open fires (SO$_2$)
• Family history	• Pets • Cigarette smoke
• Genetic	• Endotoxin exposure • Gas cookers (NO$_2$)
	• Fungal spores

Airway inflammation

Occupational factors	Outdoor environmental factors
	• Ozone • Pollens
	• Particulates • NO$_2$, SO$_2$

Airway hyper-responsiveness

Airway obstruction
↓ PEF   ↓ FEV$_1$

Symptoms	Exacerbated by
eg wheeze, cough, dyspnoea	• Infection • Smoking
	• Diet

Fig. 3. The impact of genetic and environmental factors on T_H1/T_H2 balance in asthma.
Reproduced with permission from the Annual Review of Medicine, Volume 53 © 2002 by Annual Reviews www.annualreviews.org.

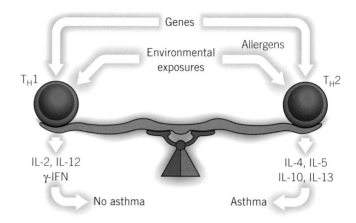

form of dysregulation of the immune cellular response, particularly involving the transition from one type of T-lymphocyte-driven immunity (T-helper 2 (T_H2) type) to another (T_H1 type) in childhood. If the child is exposed to infectious, endogenous, and environmental antigens, over time its immune system shifts toward a "healthy" T_H1/T_H2 balance (Figure 3).

Protection against immune stimulants through vaccination, frequent antibiotic use, and increased indoor activity in developed countries, may lead to a persistent T_H2 state and atopy[57] in susceptible individuals. Two areas of research support this.

1. Endotoxin exposure: one of the more interesting recent findings is that exposure to farm environments provides protection against development of atopy and asthma. Endotoxin, a component of the outer membrane of Gram-negative bacteria, is found in high concentrations in farm environments,[58] and has been shown to enhance T_H1-like immune responses.[59] It is thought that this effect of endotoxin is the reason why animal exposure protects against allergic disease.[56]

2. High levels of allergen exposure: while some exposure to an animal is needed to stimulate an allergic response, evidence indicates that higher levels of exposure may provide some protection.[60] Epidemiological studies have shown that children growing up in close contact with animals report lower prevalence of allergies, lending further support to the hygiene hypothesis.[61]

66Evidence indicates that higher levels of allergen exposure may provide some protection against atopy 99

Although breastfeeding was thought to influence development of asthma and atopy, early research evidence was conflicting, with some studies suggesting a protective effect[62–64] and some reporting an increased risk of developing asthma.[65,66] The contradictory findings can be explained by duration of follow-up in the various trials and the age at which outcomes were assessed. More definitive subsequent research concludes that breastfeeding has little protective effect in the long term.[67]

Another important influence on the T_H1/T_H2 balance is exposure to infectious agents such as viruses causing lower respiratory tract infections, for example respiratory syncytial virus (RSV).[68] Prospective studies report that RSV infections requiring hospitalization may be associated with wheezing and airway hyper-responsiveness, and possibly development of asthma.[69]

Conversely, a greater exposure to infectious agents such as measles, for example in less-developed countries, may be associated with a reduced risk of atopy.[70,71] Factors thought to be involved in the pathogenesis of asthma are shown in Figure 4.

Although useful for conceptualization, the immune mechanisms associated with atopy and cytokine imbalance (balance of T_H1/T_H2) may be oversimplified. Some studies have reported T_H1-induced reversible airway inflammation and airway hyper-responsiveness, and it is important to remember that asthma can also occur through non-allergic inflammatory mechanisms.[72,73]

> *An important influence on the T_H1/T_H2 balance is exposure to infectious agents such as viruses*

Fig. 4. Factors involved in the pathogenesis of asthma. Adapted from Holgate S T, Boushey H A, Fabbri L M (eds). Difficult Asthma (1999) with permission from Thomson Publishing Services.

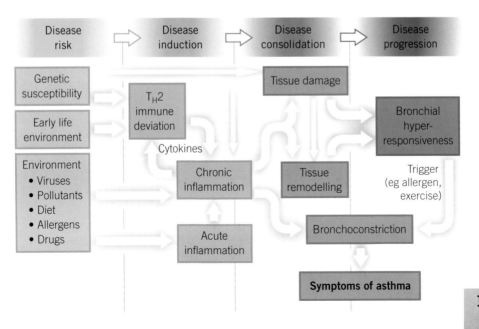

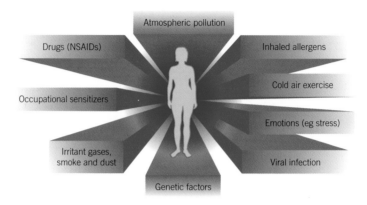

Fig. 5. Asthma triggers. Interactions between genetic and environmental factors lead to airway inflammation and hyper-responsiveness. The resulting bronchoconstriction develops in response to a variety of triggers.

For this reason, asthma should be viewed as a syndrome that occurs as a result of multiple sources of injury and repair (Figure 5) and which is mediated by a variety of mechanisms of inflammation and repair.[53] New studies investigating specific factors, timing of exposure, and how environmental and genetic factors interact will increase our understanding of the aetiology of asthma.[74]

Pathophysiology

Information on the pathogenesis of asthma has proliferated recently. Originally a model of primary smooth muscle dysfunction and reversible airway inflammation was described. Now the model includes irreversible airway remodelling.

“Changes occurring in asthma comprise acute and chronic eosinophilic and lymphocytic inflammation, smooth muscle proliferation, and epithelial and structural remodelling of the airways”

Pathophysiological mechanisms

The changes occurring in the airways of patients with asthma consist of a complex mixture of acute and chronic eosinophilic and lympho-cytic inflammation, smooth muscle proliferation, together with epithe-lial and structural remodelling and proliferation (Figure 6), and altered matrix proteins. These changes underlie airway wall narrowing and bronchial hyper-responsiveness.[75,76]

What triggers this complex pattern has recently become partially understood. Simplistically, inhaled antigens to which a patient is sen-sitive and which are not cleared by the mucociliary escalator penetrate the epithelial lining of the lung. Here they are intercepted by den-dritic cells, which present the antigen to B and T lymphocytes. A complex interaction then directs the B lymphocytes to produce allergen-specific IgE.[77]

This IgE is released into the blood and quickly binds to receptors on the surface of mast cells. Future exposure to the antigen leads to mast-cell activation. Once mast cells are activated, toxic agents, such as histamine and free radicals, are released from preformed granules to produce the "early-phase reaction",[53] which includes smooth muscle contraction, mucus secretion, vasodilatation and lumen narrowing.[75]

The release of inflammatory cytokines, such as cysteinyl leukotrienes, leads to the "late-phase reaction", where recruitment and activation of numerous cells, including eosinophils, T_H2-type CD4+ cells, macrophages, and neutrophils, ensues.[78] Once this late-phase inflammatory reaction starts, eosinophils appear to become one of the major factors interceding chronic inflammation in allergic asthma.[79] The role of allergy in asthma development is shown in Figure 7 (see page 16), while the altered cytokine balance in allergic disease is shown in Figure 8 (see page 17).[80]

Once in the airways, eosinophils release toxic granules that cause direct tissue damage, smooth muscle contraction, blood vessel leakage and lead ultimately to a vicious cycle of tissue damage and chronic recruitment of eosinophils and T_H2-type cells to the airway. Once this cycle of tissue damage is established, even without further allergen

> *Once the cycle of tissue damage is established, even without further allergen exposure, chronic recruitment of inflammatory cells may occur*

Fig. 6. Pathological changes in asthma: from broncho-constriction to airways inflammation and remodelling.
Adapted from Mol Biotech 2001;18(3):213–32 with permission from Humana Press.

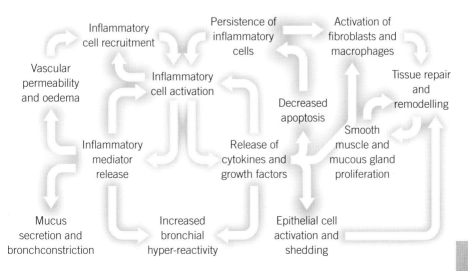

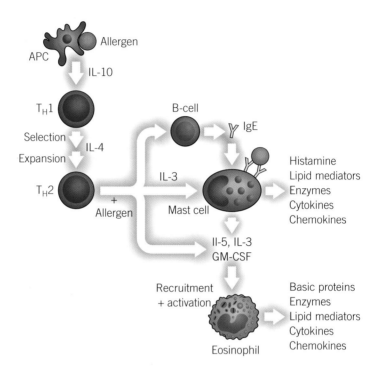

Fig. 7. The role of allergy in the development of asthma. Reprinted with permission from Nature 1999;402(6760 Suppl):B12–17 ©1999 MacMillan Magazines Limited.

exposure chronic recruitment of inflammatory cells may occur. This can be measured by production of free radicals in exhaled gas originating from neutrophils, eosinophils, and other cells involved in the inflammatory response.[81] It may be possible to measure this in the general practice setting in the future as a marker of uncontrolled inflammation.

Trials are currently underway of its usefulness in general practice to determine whether more anti-inflammatory therapy is required in patients with symptomatic asthma.

"Remodelling can be thought of as analogous to injury and healing"

Airway remodelling

It has been increasingly recognized that the chronic inflammatory process of asthma can lead to airway remodelling. Remodelling can be thought of as analogous to injury and healing.[85] After allergen exposure, injured airways tissue is repaired, restoring normal structure and function.

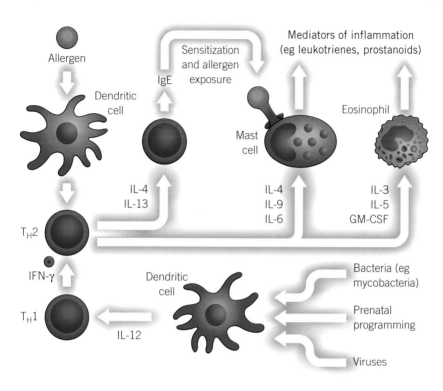

Fig. 8. The altered cytokine balance in allergic disease. Reproduced from Allergology International 2000;49: 231–36 with permission from Blackwell Publishing.

However, persistently damaged tissues may be "remodelled" through replacement by abnormal connective tissue.[75] At presentation, patients may appear to have fixed airways obstruction on a background history of asthma with no history of smoking.

The mechanism of chronic airway remodelling is not fully understood. Airway changes associated with remodelling include damage to the protective endothelial layer, laying down of collagen, smooth muscle hypertrophy, hypertrophy of the mucus glands (leading to thicker secretions) and an increase in the number of blood vessels.[53] As the bronchial walls thicken the airway lumen is reduced, heightening the bronchoconstriction resulting from bronchial hyper-responsiveness.[75]

No currently available asthma treatment has been shown to con-vincingly influence remodelling, but as our understanding of remodel-ling increases, new treatments are likely to be developed to reduce or, ultimately, prevent airway changes.

66Persistently damaged tissues may be "remodelled" through replacement by abnormal connective tissue 99

17

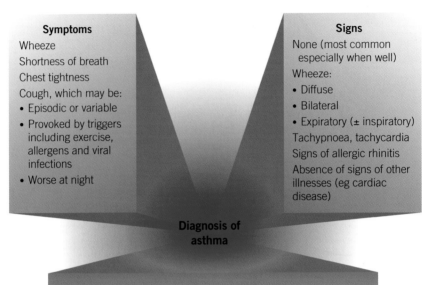

Symptoms
Wheeze
Shortness of breath
Chest tightness
Cough, which may be:
• Episodic or variable
• Provoked by triggers
including exercise,
allergens and viral
infections
• Worse at night

Signs
None (most common
especially when well)
Wheeze:
• Diffuse
• Bilateral
• Expiratory (± inspiratory)
Tachypnoea, tachycardia
Signs of allergic rhinitis
Absence of signs of other
illnesses (eg cardiac
disease)

**Diagnosis of
asthma**

Additional indicators of asthma
Personal or family history of asthma or atopy (eczema, allergic
rhinitis): up to 80% of patients with asthma will also have rhinitis
History of respiratory problems following aspirin/NSAID ingestion
or use of β-blockers (ischaemic heart disease, glaucoma)

Fig. 9. Symptoms, signs
and additional
indicators in the
diagnosis of asthma.

Diagnosis

Diagnosing asthma can be relatively straightforward when the patient
presents with typical features, but making a correct diagnosis is essential
and not all patients with asthma fulfill textbook features. Delayed or
incorrect diagnosis may lead to inadequate or inappropriate therapy,
impairment in quality of life, learnt lack of exercise and unnecessary
asthma exacerbations or even death.

Diagnosis in adults
Clinical history
The latest BTS/SIGN asthma guidelines[14] recommend practitioners
make a formal diagnosis using a mixture of good clinical history and
assessment of the features of the condition, and support this with
objective testing.

The diagnostic criteria the practitioner uses should be recorded; a
useful audit tool can be downloaded from the General Practice
Airways Group website (http://www.gpiag.org).

A person with asthma will show some or all of the symptoms and signs listed in Figure 9. Additional information that may provide evidence of asthma includes personal or family history of asthma or atopy, or a history of respiratory problems with the use of aspirin, non-steroidal anti-inflammatory drugs or ß-blockers.

Objective testing

Objective testing should ideally be carried out before starting long-term treatment. Unlike COPD, variability of airflow obstruction either in terms of forced expiratory volume in 1 second (FEV_1) using spirometry, or peak expiratory flow (PEF) using a peak flow meter, either spontaneously or in response to therapy, is characteristic of asthma (see also COPD: Diagnosis, page 64).

The latest BTS/SIGN guidelines[14] suggest that any one of the findings listed in Figure 10 is an acceptable objective measurement.

“Objective testing should be carried out before starting long-term asthma treatment”

Exercise testing

To undertake exercise testing, take a resting measurement and then ask the patient to exercise for 6 minutes. Take a further reading and then another every 10 minutes for 30 minutes. Response to exercise testing

Objective testing for asthma

- More than 20% diurnal variability on at least 3 days in a 2-week peak flow diary

- Improvement of at least 15% (and 200 ml) in the FEV_1 or 20% (and 60 l/min) in the PEF after giving a short-acting $ß_2$-agonist

- Improvement of at least 15% (and 200 ml) in the FEV_1 or 20% (and 60 l/min) in the PEF after a 2-week trial of oral prednisolone (30 mg/day) or high-dose inhaled steroid

- Deterioration of at least 15% (and 200 ml) in the FEV_1 or 20% (and 60 l/min) in the PEF after 6 minutes of vigorous exercise (for example, running)

To calculate diurnal variability (DV) insert data from the days with highest variability into the following equation:

$$DV = [(\text{highest PEF} - \text{lowest PEF}) / \text{highest PEF}] \times 100$$

Fig. 10. Acceptable objective measurements defined by BTS asthma guidelines.[14]

“Unlike COPD, variability of airflow obstruction is characteristic of asthma”

19

Fig. 11. Comparison of lung function testing using a spirometer and peak flow meter.

	Spirometry	Peak flow meter
Training required	Extensive	Minimal
Reproducibility	Very high	Low unless same PEF meter is used
Diagnosis of obstruction	Excellent	Less sensitive
Portability	Poor	Excellent. Therefore good for assessment of diurnal variability and home PEF monitoring
Cost	Relatively expensive	Cheap

will be greater if the exercise is performed in cold air. In rare cases, this test may induce an exacerbation, so appropriate treatment must be on hand.

While patients with asthma may have negative exercise tests between asthma episodes, if test results are repeatedly normal over time, especially if they are negative in the presence of symptoms, a diagnosis of asthma is unlikely. If symptoms persist and no other diagnosis appears likely, the patient should be referred for specialist challenge testing with histamine or metacholine (see Histamine/metacholine provocation tests, page 25).

❝Response to exercise testing will be greater if the exercise is performed in cold air ❞

Peak flow measurement

The correct technique is essential to ensure reliable and accurate readings with a peak flow meter or a spirometer. If the effort or technique is inadequate then the degree of airway obstruction will be overestimated. Also, the accuracy of devices varies so it is important to consistently use the same device.[83] The relative merits of spirometers and peak flow meters are listed in Figure 11. The correct method for taking a peak expiratory flow reading is shown in Figure 12.

When interpreting peak flow results, the practitioner should look at the maximal airflow the patient achieves (in litres per minute) set against a predicted normal for the patient's age, gender and race. A reduced peak flow measured against the predicted may indicate large airway obstruction, although there is substantial variation between patients.

If a change of 15% or more is demonstrated after inhalation of a bronchodilator and the patient's history suggests asthma, then diagnosis is relatively straightforward. If a 15% reversibility is not achieved then the patient should be asked to keep a peak flow chart for two weeks. A typical variable pattern is often seen, with morning dips and early evening peaks. This is known as diurnal variation (see Figure 10).

If the peak flow is low and without reversibility or diurnal variation, then a diagnosis of COPD or an alternative diagnosis is more likely. However, peak flow is not an accurate measurement for COPD because it may underestimate airway obstruction and severity and is insensitive to change.[83] But in the presence of mild-to-moderate asthma, changes in lung function may often be undetectable, especially when the patient is currently well. Exercise challenge or referral may be necessary to make a diagnosis.[84]

> **❝A typical variable pattern is often seen with peak flow measurements, with morning dips and early evening peaks❞**

Spirometry

Good-quality spirometers (examples are shown in Figures 13 and 14) are becoming less expensive and it is now common for practices to own one. Spirometry provides a more accurate assessment of lung obstruction than peak flow measurements. Substantial training is necessary to make maximal use of a spirometer, although many modern meters automatically assess the quality of readings.

The two principal measurements are the forced expiratory volume (FEV_1) – the amount of air forcibly expelled in 1 second – and the

Fig. 12. The correct method for taking a peak expiratory flow reading.

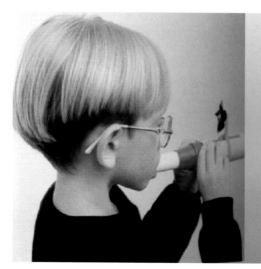

- The patient should be standing

- The peak flow meter should be held horizontally to the mouth, with the fingers free of the dial

- The patient should take the deepest inhalation possible, seal their lips around the mouthpiece and then blow out as hard and fast as they can

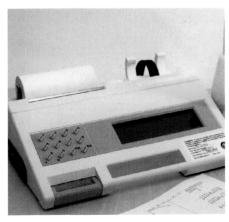

Fig. 13. Portable spirometer.

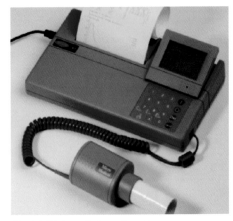

Fig. 14. High-resolution spirometer.

forced vital capacity (FVC) – the total volume of air that can be expelled from the lungs from maximum inhalation to maximum exhalation (Figure 15). The ratio of these two measurements determines the extent of airflow obstruction.

When the airways are normal 70–85% of the FVC can be exhaled in the first second. The FEV_1 is therefore normally 70–85% of the FVC. When the FEV_1/FVC ratio is reduced this indicates airflow

Fig. 15. A typical spirometer output showing the forced expiratory volume with time in a normal patient and in a patient with asthma.

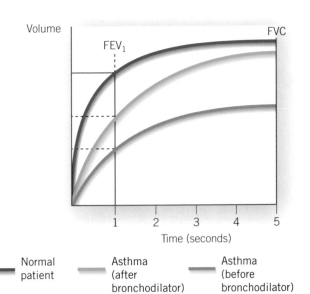

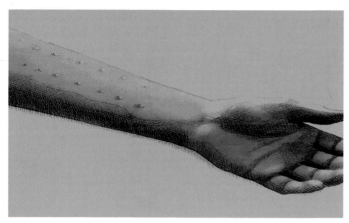

Fig. 16. Skin-prick test.

obstruction, which may be due to asthma or to COPD (see also Figure 40, page 66).

Peak expiratory flow is useful for proving asthma in younger patients and for disease monitoring. Clinic-based peak expiratory flow rates are not of much use in older patients for differentiating asthma and COPD, and ideally spirometry should be used (see Figure 11).

When choosing a spirometer it must:

- have a visual display of the flow volume loop to assess quality and reproducibility of readings
- be able to print out loops for future use
- ideally have a computer link and suitable software that enables linking of records to other patient records.

Desirable features include the ability to produce an analysis report on quality of readings obtained, and a diagnostic reporting feature.

> *Spirometry provides a more accurate assessment of lung obstruction than does peak flow measurement*

Allergy testing

Skin-prick tests (Figure 16) or specific IgE tests can detect atopy. Both are useful for establishing sensitivity or, more importantly, lack of sensitivity to specific antigens.

In a skin-prick test, small amounts of antigen extracts are placed on the flexor surface of the forearm. The tip of a stylet is used to introduce an allergen into the superficial epidermis alongside a control solution with no allergen and a control solution of histamine. A positive reaction can be seen after about 15 minutes in the form of a weal surrounded by an erythematous flare.

If properly performed, skin-prick tests yield useful confirmatory evidence for specific allergy diagnosis. However, as they are complex to perform and interpret they should be carried out by trained health professionals (for appropriate courses see Appendix 4). Scratch tests and intradermal skin tests are no longer recommended for routine use because of poor reproducibility and possible systemic reactions.

Negative and positive controls should be incuded in skin-prick tests because of the substantial variation in cutaneous reactivity between patients. Negative controls, based on diluents used to preserve the allergen vaccines, will detect the rare dermographic patient and any reaction to trauma caused by the skin test device and/or tester technique. Positive controls, usually histamine, detect suppression by medications or disease. Skin tests should be read at the peak of their reaction (usually after 15 minutes), measuring the weal and flare compared with the negative control.

Several variables may alter skin test reactions. These include quality of allergen extract, age (size of reaction is decreased in the elderly) and seasonal variation (those with a pollen allergy taking certain drugs have a depressed or absent response to skin tests for up to 6 weeks). It may not be possible to test patients with dermographism (urticaria) or widespread skin lesions.

A positive response to a skin-prick test alone does not necessarily imply the patient's symptoms are due to IgE-mediated allergy. Nevertheless, with inhaled allergens, when skin-prick test responses correlate with the clinical history, a confident diagnosis can be made.

In normal patients, levels of IgE increase from birth to adolescence and then decrease slowly and reach a plateau after age 20–30. In adults, levels over 100–150 kU/l are considered above normal. Allergic and parasitic diseases, as well as many other factors including racial variation, increase levels of total serum IgE. Therefore, a total serum IgE measurement is not predictive for allergy screening and should not be used as a diagnostic tool.

A positive response to skin tests alone does not necessarily imply that the patient's symptoms are due to IgE-mediated allergy.

In contrast, measuring allergen-specific IgE in serum is as useful as skin-prick tests. Several techniques accurately measure serum-specific IgE, including the radioallergosorbent test (RAST) and newer methods using radio- or enzyme-labelled anti-IgE. Specific IgE measurements are not influenced by drugs or skin disease. As with skin-prick tests, the presence or absence of specific IgE in the serum does not preclude symptoms, and some symptom-free people have serum-specific IgE. The cost of measuring serum-specific IgE is high and only a selected list of allergens can usually be tested.

The clinical relevance of these tests has been studied extensively and their efficiency (specificity and sensitivity) in allergy diagnosis is often over 85%. But they can define the patient only as allergic or non-allergic, and more extensive investigations may be needed if the test is positive.

Radiography

A chest radiograph may be useful to exclude other diseases and is essential in older patients with a smoking history. In children, a chest radiograph may help exclude bronchiectasis or cystic fibrosis. However, what may appear to be a normal chest x-ray does not preclude other disease processes not discernable on plain x-ray, and further investigations, such as CT scanning, may be necessary.

Histamine and metacholine provocation tests

A metacholine or histamine challenge can be a useful specialist test for patients with suspected asthma who do not demonstrate hyper-responsiveness. Under laboratory conditions, the degree of airway hyper-responsiveness can be measured by giving increasing doses of metacholine or histamine while performing serial peak flows and plotting the percentage fall.

Bronchoscopy

Referral for bronchoscopy may be considered for vocal cord dysfunction, inhalation of foreign bodies, or for suspected bronchial carcinoma.

> **" A metacholine or histamine challenge test may be useful in a patient with suspected asthma who has not demonstrated hyper-responsiveness "**

Differential diagnosis in adults

Common alternative diagnoses for asthma are listed in Figure 17.

Diagnosis in children

The most commonly reported long-term illnesses in children are conditions of the respiratory system. Two-thirds of children under age 5 consult their GP at least once a year for a respiratory condition.[1]

In children aged 5 or older the same diagnostic methods as adults can be used, however lung function is not easily measured in pre-school children and is not routinely recommended. The diagnosis of asthma in young children should be based on:

- the presence of key features (Figure 18) and the absence of features suggesting an alternative diagnosis
- an appropriate response to treatment and, if possible in milder disease, to the removal of that treatment once a stable response has been achieved
- repeated assessment of the child and evaluation of the diagnosis if management is ineffective.

The criteria used for diagnosis should be recorded.

Risk factors in children

A good history is vital for diagnosing asthma in children. Asthma is often linked to a family history of atopy. In early childhood, boys are at

25

Fig. 17. Common
differential diagnoses
for asthma.

Suspicious features	Diagnosis
• Over 40 years old • Smoker • Progressive impairment • Cough • No wheeze or minimal wheeze	COPD
• Cough • Worse at night and on bending • Heartburn or oesophageal reflux	GORD
• Smoker • Weight loss • Fatigue • Haemoptysis	Lung cancer
• Risk factors for heart disease (eg family history, hypertension, hyperlipidaemia, smoker) • Chest pain • Orthopnoea	Cardiac disease
• Sputum production often purulent and prolonged • Dysfunctional breathing not made worse with activity • No objective lung function problem	Bronchiectasis
• Progressive dyspnoea • Lack of variability • Restrictive deficit on spirometry testing	Interstitial lung disease
• Coughing when lying flat • Worse after meals	Aspiration
• Sudden onset, unilateral symptoms and signs	Foreign body
• Usually sudden onset • Dyspnoea predominant • Chest pain	Pulmonary emboli
• Dysproportionate breathlessness • Dysproportionate chest tightness • Rapid shallow and erratic breathing pattern	Dysfunctional breathing

higher risk than girls of developing asthma, although boys are more likely to "grow out" of their asthma. The reasons for this are not clear.

Differential diagnosis in children

Early age of onset, unusual patterns of symptoms, sputum production, lack of diurnal variation, associated upper respiratory symptoms, abnormal physical signs, poor control on standard inhaler therapy and unusual lung function results in older children all indicate a diagnosis other than asthma. A summary of clinical clues is shown in Figure 19.

When to refer for specialist care

Consider referring a child for specialist opinion if:
- the diagnosis is unclear
- there are unexpected clinical findings (for example, focal chest signs or radiological abnormalities)
- there is a unilateral or fixed wheeze
- there is weight loss or failure to thrive
- there is persistent cough and/or sputum production
- there is non-resolving pneumonia.

Consider a chest radiograph for patients with atypical presentations or additional symptoms such as those listed above. Conditions

66In early childhood, boys are at higher risk than girls of developing asthma 99

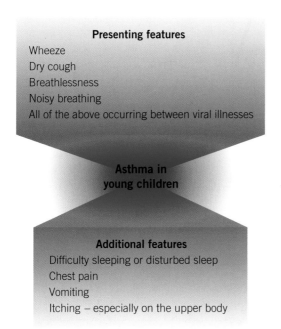

Fig. 18. Presenting and additional features of asthma in children.

Presenting features
Wheeze
Dry cough
Breathlessness
Noisy breathing
All of the above occurring between viral illnesses

Asthma in young children

Additional features
Difficulty sleeping or disturbed sleep
Chest pain
Vomiting
Itching – especially on the upper body

in children that are often confused with asthma are listed in Figure 20.

Occupational asthma

Occupational asthma is the most common industrial lung disease in the developing world[85] and between 1990 and 1997 over 6500 cases were reported to the "Surveillance of Work-related and Occupational Respiratory Disease" (SWORD) reporting system.[86] SWORD is a national surveillance programme that produces monthly reports on new cases of occupational respiratory disease to raise the profile of potentially hazardous sensitizers for further investigation.

Although occupational asthma has many definitions, all of them include core features such as variable airflow limitation that is related

Fig. 19. "Typical" presentation of asthma in young children. The triggers to exacerbations may be viral illnesses, exercise, animals, other aeroallergens, aerosols, perfumes and emotions. Adapted from Paed Respir Rev 2002;3(2):148–53 with permission from Elsevier Ltd.

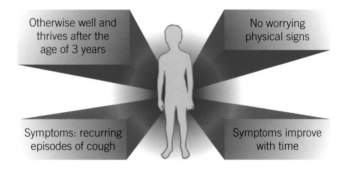

Otherwise well and thrives after the age of 3 years

No worrying physical signs

Symptoms: recurring episodes of cough

Symptoms improve with time

to work, specific airway hyper-responsiveness (if of allergic origin), and non-specific airway hyper-responsiveness.[87]

Whether identified or not, the causal agent must be encountered only in the workplace, negating triggers such as exercise or cold air. Occupational asthma is divided into two types, allergic and non-allergic (Figure 21).

The many factors that influence development of occupational asthma include:

• exposure: type, intensity, frequency and magnitude of the exposure
• mode of employment: different levels of use of causal agents in specific jobs
• geographical location: clustering of occupational asthma cases and industries
• industrial factors: different working conditions and industrial processes
• personal factors: atopy and smoking behaviour.

Condition	Comment
"Viral-associated wheeze"	If symptoms occur only with viral infections, the child is entirely well between episodes,and there is no family history of atopy or asthma, the child is likely to have a self-limiting illness. Prophylactic asthma treatment has not been shown to work for these children
Gastro-oesophageal reflux	If respiratory symptoms are prominent when lying down, especially if associated with excessive vomiting in a young child (typically at night), consider gastro-oesophageal reflux
Cystic fibrosis and other causes of bronchiectasis	Asthmatic children under age 8 do not cough up sputum, and it is uncommon in older children. Therefore, any child who produces sputum merits full investigation as a diagnosis of asthma is usually untenable. Other associated symptoms include failure to thrive
Primary ciliary dyskinesia syndrome	A runny nose is common in infants over 4 months, but a runny nose from birth strongly suggests primary ciliary dyskinesia syndrome
Upper airway disease	Post-nasal drip can be easily confused with asthma, and the two often co-exist. These children cough at night (when lying flat) and may produce "sputum," but this is simply recycling of the post-nasal drip discharge. Snoring is another sign
Structural airway disease	Symptoms from the first few days of life imply a structural defect that demands full investigation
Endobronchial foreign body	Sudden-onset and one-sided symptoms and signs may indicate an endobronchial foreign body
Non-organic symptoms	In vocal cord dysfunction the vocal cords adduct instead of abduct during inspiration. Patients are asymptomatic at night and have a habit cough. This is more common in older children and teenagers

Fig. 20. Conditions in children often confused with asthma.

Allergic occupational asthma

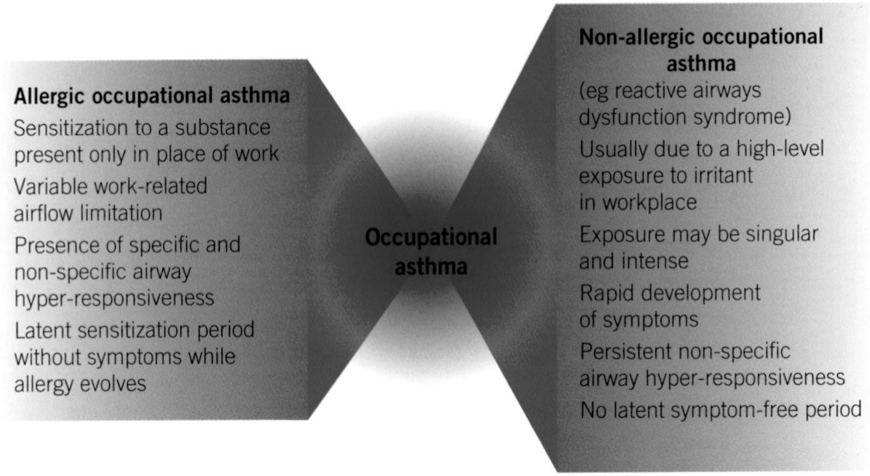

Sensitization to a substance present only in place of work

Variable work-related airflow limitation

Presence of specific and non-specific airway hyper-responsiveness

Latent sensitization period without symptoms while allergy evolves

Occupational asthma

Non-allergic occupational asthma

(eg reactive airways dysfunction syndrome)

Usually due to a high-level exposure to irritant in workplace

Exposure may be singular and intense

Rapid development of symptoms

Persistent non-specific airway hyper-responsiveness

No latent symptom-free period

Fig. 21. Occupational asthma is divided into two types, allergic and non-allergic.

Causal agents

Over 200 agents have been shown to be positively associated with occupational asthma.[85] They can originate from animals, insects, bacterial enzymes, woods, plants, marine life, drugs and chemicals. The most common culprits are listed in Figure 22. Finding a specific cause can be much harder than establishing a relationship between asthma symptoms and the workplace.

Diagnosing occupational asthma

A diagnosis of occupational asthma should be considered in any patient with adult-onset asthma, and in patients experiencing breathlessness or other respiratory symptoms who work in industries with a high risk of occupational asthma. All patients with a suspicious history should be referred for prompt specialist assessment. Early diagnosis is very important because it allows prompt treatment, early removal of triggering factor and improves the prognosis.[88,89]

66All patients with a suspicious history should be referred for prompt assessment for occupational asthma 99

History

A documented relationship between the development of symptoms and attendance at the workplace should be determined. It is important to remember that in more severe disease a weekend away from work may not be enough to alleviate symptoms, and the relationship may only be apparent with longer holidays.

Specialist investigations

To confirm a work–asthma relationship, serial measurements of peak expiratory flow (PEF) are usually necessary. These are taken every 2 hours from waking until sleeping including during the work period.

If the validity of PEF recording is suspect, measurements of non-specific responsiveness with metacholine and/or histamine can be made after a period of work exposure and after a period of non-exposure (see Histamine/metacholine provocation tests, page 25).

Specific immunological testing, either with a RAST test or skin-prick test, may reveal a causal agent. Bronchial challenge testing is considered the gold standard for diagnosing occupational asthma.[90] Exposure must be controlled carefully to prevent violent reaction. Reaction time can vary dramatically, peaking in a few minutes to 4–8 hours.

> **"Workers should not be told to leave their job until the diagnosis has been confirmed"**

Management of occupational asthma

Workers should not be told to leave their job until the diagnosis has been confirmed. Once confirmation is received immediate removal from the offending agent is essential. Owing to the potentially life-changing nature of a definitive diagnosis, the patient should seek employer compensation and the employer should offer advice and support. The industry should be made aware of the hazardous agent, identify and survey other employees for new cases and seek alternative processes that do not involve use of the substance.[14]

Prognosis

Avoiding exposure does not always stop symptoms; indeed some patients suffer symptoms for months or years after the last exposure. The longer the exposure and duration of symptoms before diagnosis

Fig. 22. Main causes of occupational asthma.

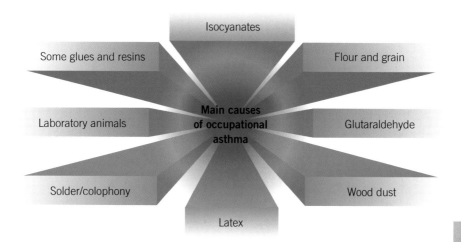

the worse the prognosis,[91] especially in those exposed for more than 1 year,[92] so early diagnosis is paramount.

Treatment of asthma

The aims of asthma management[14] are shown in Figure 23.

Non-pharmacological therapy

There is increasing interest in non-drug approaches to improving asthma or even preventing the disease entirely. We will first examine approaches to preventing asthma development.

Asthma prevention

Much of the data on asthma prevention is inconclusive but it is worth recommending smoking cessation. Other interventions, such as immunotherapy and probiotic use, look promising but more research is needed. Other preventative measures include:

> *Clear benefits have been shown for smoking cessation, weight reduction (in the obese) and allergen avoidance in the treatment of asthma*

- allergen avoidance: many studies are underway or have recently looked at this as a method of asthma prevention. To date the evidence remains unclear and no firm recommendations can be made that might help to prevent asthma development
- immunotherapy: data in allergic rhinitis suggest that this may be of benefit especially in patients with severe rhinitis unresponsive to therapy and especially in patients who are allergic to one allergen
- breastfeeding: while important for many other reasons, protective effects in asthma remain unproven
- dietary manipulation: no clear evidence from intervention studies has emerged, although many interesting studies are underway including trials of fish oil supplements in pregnancy
- microbial exposure: the *"hygiene hypothesis"* (see page 11) has led to trials of probiotics; clear results are awaited
- smoking avoidance: while not shown to prevent asthma development, smoking avoidance in pregnancy is associated with a reduction in wheezing illness in the first 3 years of life
- avoiding air pollution: while theoretically attractive, avoiding air pollution has not been shown to reduce rates of asthma development.

Non-pharmacological asthma treatment

There is much more evidence for the efficacy of non-pharmacological measures in *treatment* than *prevention*, with clear benefits shown for smoking cessation, weight reduction (in the obese) and allergen avoidance (provided adequate reductions take place). Immunotherapy and physiotherapy may play a role in the future. The benefits of complementary therapy are not proven.

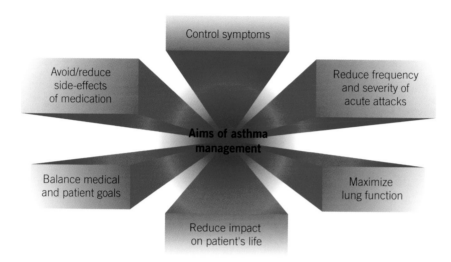

Fig. 23. Aims of asthma management.

Allergen avoidance

There is substantially more evidence for the effectiveness of allergen avoidance in asthma treatment than in asthma prevention. The limiting factor with some allergens is the difficulty of reducing allergen load enough to produce improvement. When an allergen has been *proven* to worsen asthma, and when exposure can be reduced adequately (such as allergy to a pet), this seems very worthwhile. However, reducing levels of house dust mites enough to make a difference requires enormous commitment and expense, and in general is not recommended.

Immunotherapy (desensitization)

There is increasing evidence for the efficacy of immunotherapy in treating asthma and allergic rhinitis. However, there is little evidence for its effectiveness compared with existing asthma therapy. Moreover, immunotherapy should only be undertaken where full resuscitation facilities are available. It is possible that advances in administering immunotherapy, such as the use of the sublingual route, may bring this therapy back into the mainstream of asthma management in the UK.

Dietary manipulation

No studies have confirmed the value of dietary manipulation, except for weight loss in the obese.

"Immunotherapy and physiotherapy may play a role in asthma treatment in the future"

Avoiding exposure to cigarette smoke

This is very beneficial in patients with asthma and can be expected to reduce severity, increase patient response to inhaled corticosteroids and slow progression or development of COPD. This should always be recommended and the appropriate psychological and pharmacological support provided.

66No studies have confirmed the value of dietary manipulation, except for weight loss in the obese 99

Reducing air pollution

Data on the effect of avoiding exposure to air pollution are unclear, although it appears worthwhile during strenuous activity and exercise in patients with severe disease on days with severe atmospheric pollution.

Breathing exercises and Buteyko technique

Very recent research suggests that some asthma patients with evidence of dysfunctional breathing may benefit from physiotherapy. This may affect up to one third of women and one fifth of men with asthma.[93] It appears that up to one half benefit from breathing retraining in terms of improvements in quality of life.[94] More research is needed but it is a promising therapy for the future.[94]

Other complementary therapy

There is no clear evidence for the benefit of any herbal therapy, acupuncture, air ionizers, homeopathy, hypnosis or manual therapy in asthma.[14]

Pharmacological therapy

66The main aim of pharmacological therapy is to manage asthma so that symptoms are prevented, lifestyle limitation is avoided and best lung function is achieved with minimal side-effects 99

The main aim of pharmacological therapy is to manage asthma so that symptoms are prevented, lifestyle limitation is avoided and best lung function is achieved with minimal side-effects. It is important to consider potential side-effects when making treatment decisions and to achieve the optimal balance between disease control and medication level. The patient's view is fundamental to agreeing targets of asthma management.

The major drug classes used to manage patients with asthma are shown in Figure 24.

Inhaled corticosteroids (beclomethasone, budesonide, fluticasone, mometasone)

Inhaled corticosteroids (ICS) have become the mainstay of treatment for persistent asthma because of their significant clinical benefits and minimal major systemic side-effects at low doses. They work by reducing the airways inflammation associated with asthma

LABAs may also be used to prevent exercise-induced bronchospasm. Salmeterol and formoterol produce a similar duration of bronchodilation, but formoterol has a more rapid onset of action than salmeterol, which may be useful in some patients to provide occasional symptom relief.

Side-effects
Systemic side-effects, such as cardiovascular stimulation and tremor, are much rarer than with oral therapy.

Fig. 25. Mechanisms of action of inhaled long-acting ß-agonists.

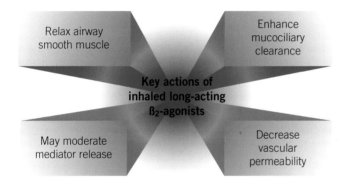

Relax airway smooth muscle

Enhance mucociliary clearance

Key actions of inhaled long-acting ß$_2$-agonists

May moderate mediator release

Decrease vascular permeability

Combination inhalers of steroids and long-acting ß$_2$-agonists (Seretide, Symbicort)

Because adding an inhaled LABA to an ICS may have a greater efficacy than increasing the dose of ICS, fixed combination inhalers have been developed. The two currently available preparations are Seretide (fluticasone propionate plus salmeterol) and Symbicort (budesonide plus formoterol).

Clinical trials have shown that fixed combination inhalers have a comparable efficacy to combinations of the individual inhalers. In addition, the fixed combination inhalers are likely to have advantages in terms of compliance and ensure that the LABA is always accompanied by an ICS. In some circumstances, the combination may be less expensive than administering the two drugs separately.

As a result of these factors combination inhalers have been widely adopted in clinical practice.

❝Fixed combination inhalers are likely to have compliance advantages and ensure that the LABA is always accompanied by an ICS ❞

39

Oral long-acting ß₂-agonists (salbutamol and terbutaline in sustained-release tablets, and bambuterol)

Oral LABAs have frequent side-effects, including tachycardia, anxiety, skeletal muscle tremor, headache and, more rarely, hypokalaemia. They are therefore limited to add-on treatment in patients with moderate-to-severe asthma who are unresponsive to other add-on therapy and to increased ICS. They appear to have similar effectiveness to sustained-release theophylline.

Leukotriene receptor antagonists (montelukast, zafirlukast)

LTRAs selectively block the leukotriene cysLT1 receptor, thereby inhibiting the bronchoconstrictive and inflammatory effects of the leukotrienes. Leukotrienes are inflammatory mediators heavily implicated in asthma pathophysiology, and do not appear to be blocked by inhaled steroids.[260] LTRAs have a rapid onset of action and are given orally.

Limited trials in patients with mild asthma suggest that the control achieved with montelukast is comparable to that achieved with ICS. LTRAs may be particularly useful in people with predominant exercise symptoms or post-viral symptoms, especially the very young or those who will not, or cannot, take ICS.

In people with moderate or severe disease ICS are clearly superior to LTRAs and remain the first choice anti-inflammatory therapy. However, for people with moderate asthma, there is substantial evidence that montelukast, as add-on therapy to corticosteroids, increases asthma control, reduces asthma exacerbations and improves the level of symptomatic relief to the same extent as increasing the dose of ICS.[102, 103]

A recent study of LTRAs has shown comparable reductions in exacerbations and improvements in asthma symptoms to adding a LABA, and greater reductions in eosinophils, although less improvement in lung function.[255] As with all asthma therapy there is a variation in response, with some patients clearly having a more marked response than others. While there are no absolute predictors, patients with exercise symptoms, post-viral symptoms or co-existing rhinitis may benefit most.

66LTRAs may be particularly useful in people with predominant exercise symptoms or post-viral symptoms, especially the very young or those who will not, or cannot, take ICS 99

Side-effects

Side-effects appear to be rare, although liver enzyme abnormalities have been reported with unlicensed doses of zafirlukast.

Oral xanthines (theophylline, aminophylline)

This drug class is given orally and is one of the oldest used in asthma. Oral xanthines appear to have two mechanisms of action.

- At low doses they seem to have a limited influence on chronic airway inflammation, although the mechanism is unclear.
- At higher doses they produce bronchodilator effects, which are thought to be related to phophodiesterase inhibition.

Sustained-release theophylline and aminophylline are used principally as an add-on treatment in patients with moderate-to-severe persistent asthma. They are not recommended as first choice because of difficulties in titrating individual dose and the high occurrence of potentially serious side-effects at high serum concentrations, including seizures, tachycardia, and arrhythmias. Serum levels should be measured if these drugs are used.

Absorption and metabolism may also be affected by many factors, including febrile illnesses. Nausea and vomiting are the most common side-effects.

66Oral xanthines are one of the oldest drug classes used in the treatment of asthma 99

Cromones (sodium cromoglicate, nedocromil sodium)

Sodium cromoglicate and nedocromil sodium are given via inhalation. Their exact mechanisms of action are poorly understood. They appear to partly inhibit IgE-mediated mediator release from mast cells as well as suppressing some mediator-related effects on other inflammatory cells, including eosinophils. While this suggests that cromones have anti-inflammatory effects, this has not been clearly proven in long-term clinical trials.

Trials have shown that while these drugs have small effects on symptoms and frequency of exacerbations, they are significantly less effective than ICS. They now play a minor role in asthma management as an alternative to ICS in adults with mild disease (who will not or cannot take ICS), and as an add-on therapy when other therapeutic options have been tried and failed. The advantage of cromones is that they produce only minimal side-effects, such as occasional coughing when inhaling the powder formulation. However, some patients dislike the taste of nedocromil sodium. Another drawback is that sodium cromoglicate must be taken four times a day.

The stepwise approach

International and British guidelines recommend a stepwise approach to managing asthma symptoms. The aim is to achieve control early by starting on the appropriate step and maintaining this control by stepping treatment up or down according to patient need. The initial step chosen should reflect symptom severity.

Before changing treatment, aim to identify and eliminate avoidable trigger factors and assess treatment compliance, including correct inhaler technique.

41

Detecting poorly controlled patients

Detecting poorly controlled patients in general practice is not as easy as it seems. Many will not attend for review and, in those that do, poor control manifested as substantial lifestyle limitation may remain undetected unless the right questions are asked, since many patients tend to regard their asthma symptoms as normal.[95, 96]

There are two key elements in detecting poorly controlled patients:

1. Using routinely recorded data: if the prescribing records are examined, many of these patients will have high ß_2-agonist use as described in Step 2 (using more than one inhaler in 6 weeks – see page 43). These patients should be invited for review or offered a telephone appointment. Telephone appointments are now recognized as an effective way of increasing the number of patients reviewed,[97] and will help to meet the target of patient review included in the new contract for GPs in the UK (see Appendix 2).

2. Optimize the patient consultation: much work has shown that patients with uncontrolled asthma do not recognize it as such, as they have become used to it. It is therefore key to explore symptoms and lifestyle limitation – possibly using the Royal College of Physicians' three questions as prompts as recommended by current BTS/SIGN asthma guidelines (Figure 26).

> **"Detecting poorly controlled patients in general practice is not as easy as it seems"**

Step 1: Mild intermittent asthma

Managing mild intermittent asthma with periodic and occasional short-acting ß_2-agonists (SABAs) alone is recommended by national and international guidelines. Patients who are suitable for this minimal level of management should have symptoms relating to only a few scenarios; for example, symptoms linked to exercise, or exercise alongside allergen challenge (such as during the hayfever season). These symptoms should be mild at worst and provide no more than minor inconvenience at work or school.

When taking a history from such patients, it is important that they are questioned carefully. Do they truly feel well between episodes? Is their lifestyle limited or have their symptoms become habitual? Objective monitoring of lung function and symptoms when the patient is well will help to ensure their asthma is truly intermittent.

SABAs relieve the symptoms of bronchoconstriction by stimulating ß_2-adrenoreceptors in the smooth muscle of the airways, causing smooth muscle relaxation and bronchodilation. The onset is rapid, within minutes, and the bronchodilator effect lasts around 3–5 hours.

Because SABAs give only temporary symptom relief and cannot control the underlying inflammatory process, excessive inhaler use may indicate poor control. Patients who appear to be using high levels of

SABAs should be reviewed. The threshold for this is debated. Nevertheless, for a patient being treated for what is apparently mild intermittent asthma the threshold should be low and certainly no higher than one relief inhaler per month.

Step 2: Regular preventer therapy

For adults with persistent asthma or more severe intermittent asthma, significant airway inflammation is presumed. The most effective agents for treating this inflammation, improving lung function and reducing symptoms and exacerbations are inhaled corticosteroids (ICS) (for example, budesonide, beclomethasone dipropionate and

❝Excessive inhaler use may indicate poor control of the patient's asthma ❞

Three key questions to detect poorly controlled patients	
Question 1	In the last week how many days have you had difficulty sleeping because of your asthma symptoms (including cough)? Score from 0 to 7 and record in the notes
Question 2	In the last week how many days have you had your usual asthma symptoms during the day (cough, wheeze, chest tightness or breathlessness)?
Question 3	In the last week how many days has your asthma interfered with your usual activities (eg, housework, work, school)?

Fig. 26. Detecting poorly controlled patients. Three key questions for determining and assessing extent of symptoms and lifestyle limitation.

fluticasone propionate) provided that they are taken regularly by patients.

Guidelines suggest regular preventer medication should be introduced in patients who have experienced recent exacerbations, nocturnal symptoms, impaired lung function or who use SABAs more than two or three times a day (using one relief inhaler every 6 weeks or more). In patients who previously used relief treatment once a day, research shows a substantial benefit in symptom control by introducing regular preventer medication.[98]

A reasonable starting dose in adults is 400 mcg (200 mcg in children) but doses must be specifically tailored to achieve optimal control for each individual. Half these doses should be used for fluticasone, mometasone and the hydrofluoroalkane formulation of beclomethasone (Qvar).

It is essential that patients understand the need for daily, regular use of these prophylactic medications to achieve treatment goals and, although initially twice-daily dosing is recommended once control is established, once-daily dosing (at the same total daily dose) may aid adherence.

> *It is important to review patients regularly to achieve optimal disease management with minimal side-effects*

It is important to review asthma patients regularly to achieve optimal disease management with minimal side-effects. Stepping up or, equally importantly, stepping down treatment to the required dose is essential. Regular daily doses should not normally exceed 800 mcg in adults and 400 mcg in children.

Side-effects such as skin bruising and cataracts may be associated with high doses of ICS, along with bone mineral density loss and osteoporosis, especially in postmenopausal women and those with inactivity related to severe disease.[99]

Local side-effects, including dysphonia and oropharyngeal candidiasis, may occur at any dose and are relatively common. These may be improved by changing the patient's inhaler device or using a spacer. However, patients often require a reduction in the dose of inhaled steroid.

In children, total daily doses of 400 mcg or more have been associated with short-term growth suppression and, more rarely, adrenal suppression.[100,101] While growth suppression is likely to be short-term, children's height should be monitored regularly. Children requiring more than 400 mcg/day on a regular basis should have a specialist review. Any child presenting with a decreased level of consciousness should be checked for adrenal insufficiency.

Other preventer therapies may be used when patients are unable or unwilling to take ICS, although every effort should be made to persuade patients with moderately severe disease (impaired lung function, history of exacerbations or daily symptoms, especially nocturnal awakenings) to take ICS even if in low doses and in conjunction with other therapy. Other preventer therapies recognized by current UK guidelines include leukotriene receptor antagonists and theophylline.

Many patients have substantial fears about taking regular ICS and these need to be explored fully before starting therapy or if a patient appears not to be taking ICS as planned.

Step 3: Add-on therapy
Many patients are controlled suboptimally when taking ICS at maximal doses recommended for Step 2 (800 mcg adults, 400 mcg

children), with up to one-half of patients complaining of significant symptoms and lifestyle limitation.[95,96]

A major cause of suboptimal control may be poor adherence or poor inhaler technique. A review of both of these issues and possibly a change in inhaler device or a renewed commitment by the patient to take their ICS more regularly may improve asthma control. Coexisting rhinitis should also be considered because this may lead to significant symptoms and worse asthma control in its own right.

Before increasing therapy one should ask:

* Does the patient have asthma?
* Is the patient taking his or her current asthma therapy as planned? (If not try to find out why, and encourage the patient to take therapy or change therapy)
* Is the patient able to use their inhaler properly? (If not, see if they are amenable to training or change the device)
* Does the patient have uncontrolled concomitant rhinitis?
* Does the patient have concomitant dysfunctional breathing?

If poor control persists after checking and resolving other causes, add-on therapy options are recommended. The correct dose of ICS to add-on as supplementary asthma therapy cannot be stated clearly, as patients seem to differ in their response to asthma medications. As a rule, patients should not be increased beyond 800 mcg of ICS (400 mcg in children) without a trial of add-on therapy first. If one trial of add-on therapy does not work, another should usually be tried; if partial benefit occurs it is worth a continued trial of this therapy and to increase the ICS to 800 mcg if not already done.

The current first choice add-on therapy is a long-acting β_2-agonist (LABA) such as salmeterol or formoterol. LABAs (for example salmeterol or formoterol) improve lung function and reduce symptoms and exacerbations in many patients who are uncontrolled on ICS. They have a duration of action of at least 12 hours. They may either be given in an additional stand-alone inhaler or as a combination inhaler, which contains an ICS and a LABA. A 1-month trial of therapy should usually establish whether a clinically important benefit has been found.

If poor control persists after checking and resolving other causes, add-on therapy options are recommended

If this addition does not improve asthma control, it is appropriate to undertake a trial of another add-on therapy, such as an LTRA (for example montelukast or zafirlukast) or a combination of theophylline and a slow-release oral β_2-agonist. Emerging evidence suggests that LTRAs might be used earlier in those with significant activity or exercise problems, concomitant rhinitis and in children.

LTRAs work by blocking the effects of cysteinyl leukotrienes (previously known as slow-reacting substance of anaphylaxis) in the

45

airways. They improve lung function, symptoms and reduce exacerbations. Recent research reports that, as an add-on therapy to 800 mcg daily ICS, montelukast has a faster onset of action and may reduce risk of side-effects compared with doubling the daily ICS dose to 1600 mcg.[102]

LTRAs have also been shown to be as effective as add-on therapy to ICS in a vast variety of doses,[103] and are as effective as LABAs.[255] They appear to be most effective in those with activity symptoms or with concomitant rhinitis.

Theophyllines and slow-release oral β_2-agonists improve lung function and symptoms but are associated with more frequent side-effects than LTRAs or LABAs. Cromone add-on therapy is of marginal benefit and add-on anticholinergics are generally of no value.

> *Children who are inadequately controlled at Step 4 or who require doses of ICS over 400 mcg should be referred to a specialist"*

Step 4: Persistent poor control
If control is still inadequate for patients taking 800 mcg ICS plus add-on therapy as described in Step 3, a trial of the following is recommended:
* increase ICS to 2000 mcg daily (800 mcg children aged 5–12 years)
* give add-on LTRAs
* give add-on theophylline
* give slow-release oral β_2-agonists – use with caution if the patient is also taking LABAs.

If any of these trials is ineffective:
* in the case of ICS titrate to the original dose
* for add-on therapies stop the medication
* consider referral to specialist care, especially in children who are inadequately controlled at Step 4 or who require doses of more than 400 mcg ICS.

Step 5: Continuous or frequent use of oral steroid
Short courses of oral corticosteroids (for example, prednisolone) are commonly used to treat an asthma exacerbation, but long-term oral corticosteroids may be required to control chronic, severe asthma. Oral corticosteroid doses should be titrated as much as possible to control symptoms and reduce unpleasant side-effects. Patients taking long-term oral steroids, especially for more than 3 months should be referred to specialist care and monitored for:
* high blood pressure
* diabetes mellitus
* osteoporosis
* growth retardation
* cataract formation.
Patients should be given side-effect advice and a steroid card.

Oral steroid-sparing regimes

Oral steroids are strongly associated with side-effects, therefore steroid-sparing regimes should be considered wherever possible. ICS up to doses of 2000 mcg daily (do not exceed 1000 mcg in children aged 5–12 years without careful consideration) are recommended to reduce and eliminate oral steroid use over time. A 6-week trial of either LTRAs or theophyllines may be undertaken to monitor improvements in symptoms, lung function or reduction in oral steroid use. Medication should be stopped if no improvements are made.

"Many patients are not seen for review, denying them the opportunity of reducing medication"

Stepping down other medications

Many patients are not seen for regular review, denying them the opportunity of reducing medication. For these patients, over-treatment and avoidable side-effects can result. Once the asthma is controlled, the dose of ICS especially should be reduced in carefully monitored patients. Patients should be maintained at the lowest possible dose, but reduction should be slow because deterioration rates differ between individuals. Guidelines recommend ICS dose reductions of 25–50% every 3 months. The choice of type and rate of medication reduction must be based on patient preference, clinical benefit and side-effects.

Exercise and asthma

Exercise-induced bronchoconstriction can develop within minutes of beginning vigorous exercise; however, this response appears to resolve within 30 minutes followed by a refractory period of about 2 hours when further exercise does not provoke bronchoconstriction.

Exercise-induced asthma can be an indication of poorly controlled disease and regular prophylactic treatment with ICS should be considered. Patients can be advised to "warm up" and also to take SABAs immediately prior to exercise, although this may not always be feasible in children. Other medications that protect against exercise-induced asthma include ICS, LABAs, theophyllines, LTRAs, cromones and ß$_2$-agonist tablets.

"Exercise-induced broncho-constriction can develop within minutes of beginning vigorous exercise"

LABAs and LTRAs provide more prolonged protection than SABAs, although a degree of tolerance to this action has been reported with LABAs, which is not seen with LTRA use. Use of such agents may be particularly useful in children and adults with symptoms brought on by exercise or activity, despite taking background ICS. It is of fundamental importance that patients should not lead lives limited by their asthma. Indeed, there is good evidence that asthma is no barrier to sportsmanship since 67 athletes with asthma won medals in the 1984 Olympic games.[104]

Devices for drug delivery
Inhalers

Most asthma medication is administered via inhalation to the site of the disease mechanism in the lungs. Many different inhaler delivery systems are available (Figure 27), including self-actuated pressurized metered-dose inhalers (MDIs) breath-activated inhalers (BAIs) and dry powder inhalers (DPIs). MDIs use propellants to deliver medication to the lungs. Until recently, propellants were exclusively chlorofluorocarbon-driven but are now being replaced with hydrofluoroalkanes. Each system has advantages and disadvantages with respect to drug deposition, ease of use and cost.

Acceding to a general lack of evidence, the current BTS/SIGN guidelines generally report equivalence between MDI with spacer, BAI

Fig. 27. The many different types of asthma inhalers.

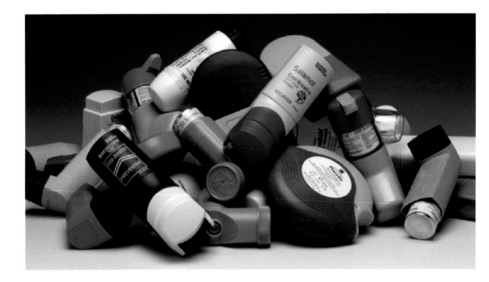

and DPI, although they acknowledge that patients may be unwilling to carry a spacer. Guidelines suggest that selection of inhaler should be based primarily on local cost and patient preference, although assessment of inhaler technique by a health care professional is also recommended.

MDIs are the most widely prescribed devices in most countries, including the UK, although technique is often reported to be deficient.[105, 106] Poor co-ordination between breathing and firing, and hasty inspiration are common problems, and drug delivery to the lung can vary between 7% and 20%.[107]

A recent systematic review surprisingly concluded that MDIs are as clinically effective as all other inhaler types,[108, 109] although this has been challenged by a recent "real-life" observational general practice study, which reported fewer oral steroid prescriptions, fewer GP consultations for asthma, and better overall asthma control in children and adults using BAIs compared with MDIs.[110] At present MDIs should be used when the patient can clearly demonstrate adequate inhaler technique.

66 MDIs are the most widely prescribed devices in most countries, despite deficient metered dose inhaler technique 99

Spacers

Spacer devices (for example the Aerochamber™, Babyhaler™, Volumatic™ and Nebuhaler™) are useful for almost all asthmatic patients but are particularly beneficial in children under age 7, and patients taking ICS who are prone to oral thrush or dysphonia. The spacer eliminates the need for co-ordination between actuating the MDI and inhaling. It can also be adapted for young children, toddlers and even infants by adding a facemask.[111]

It is important to ensure the spacer selected is appropriate for the inhaler device it will be used with. Single actuations of the MDI into the spacer followed by inhalation are the recommended method of use, with minimal delay between actuation and inhalation. Tidal breathing is equally effective as single deep breaths.

Electrostatic charges in plastic spacers drastically reduce drug delivery.[112,113] Detergent is the best anti-static agent for spacers; therefore spacers should be washed with detergent once monthly and left to dry in the air, wiping only the mouthpiece free of detergent before use. The major drawback of spacers is that they are bulky and often not used by patients.

Nebulizers

The commonest indication for using a nebulizer is for emergency treatment and where large doses of inhaled drugs are needed. Using an MDI with a spacer is at least as effective as a nebulizer for treating mild-to-moderate asthma in children under age 2, and there is no evidence that nebulizers are superior to MDIs and spacers for delivering ICS in chronic asthma. An MDI with a spacer helps achieve a high-lung and low-extra-pulmonary dose and can perform better than a nebulizer.[111] Additionally, only high-dose formulations of nebulized drugs are licensed, making nebulizer use more appropriate for acute asthma.[14]

In a study comparing previous nebulizer use with spacer use in 73 children with acute asthma, 84% of parents said the spacer was easier to use, 77% said the spacer was better tolerated by their child, and 84% said that, overall, they preferred the spacer.[114]

66 Nebulizers are most commonly used in emergency treatment where large doses of inhaled drugs are needed 99

The 1997 British Thoracic Society guidelines on nebulizer assessment and use[115] recommend that nebulized bronchodilators be used only in chronic severe asthma for the relief of symptoms at Step 4 of the asthma guidelines (see page 46).

Use of nebulized corticosteroids for reducing steroid dependence should only be undertaken after a review by a respiratory specialist.

66Patient's attitudes impact on their illness, affecting their coping skills and adherence to treatment regimes 99

Psychological and social issues in asthma

Since most day-to-day disease management is undertaken by the patient, the overall success of treatment relies on patient factors. Managing the psychological elements of asthma is interwoven with more tangible patient factors such as inhaler technique and adherence to treatment regimes.

Asthma may be affected by psychological factors [116,117] suggesting the need for a holistic approach to the treatment of asthma that takes into account clinical and psychological aspects of the disease.

Psychosocial factors are strongly associated with asthma mortality and near-fatal exacerbations. Near fatal asthma attacks are related to lack of prompt action by patients and their relatives.[118] Moreover, there appears to be an association between psychiatric and asthma morbidity, with the experience of a near-fatal attack increasing the denial of health or psychiatric problems.[119]

The adverse behavioural or psychosocial features associated with the risk of near-fatal or fatal asthma are listed in Figure 28. These are derived from the BTS/SIGN guidelines on managing asthma.

Patient's attitudes therefore impact on their illness, affecting their coping skills and adherence to treatment regimes.

Successful self-management of asthma is important, and recognition of psychosocial aspects of the disease have resulted in the integration of cognitive-behavioural therapy,[120] and group and individual counselling,[121] with educational packages about asthma self-management. Other psychoeducation techniques have incorporated autogenic therapy[122] and relaxation therapy.[116] Evidence comparing the relative effectiveness of these interventions is needed to support referral decisions.[123]

Nevertheless, psychoeducational programmes that integrate relaxation and behavioural techniques have reported improved health outcomes for adults with asthma.[124]

In children and adolescents, specific psychological factors (for example anxiety, external reinforcement of symptomatic behaviour, faulty symptom attribution, lack of knowledge, poor self-efficacy and a desire for autonomy) may have a negative impact on the symptoms and management of asthma. Parental mental health problems or poor coping skills may also have a negative influence in children.[125]

Features associated with fatal or near-fatal exacerbations

- Non-compliance with treatment or monitoring
- Failure to attend appointments
- Self-discharge from hospital
- Psychosis, depression, other psychiatric illness or self-harm
- Current or recent tranquillizer use
- Denial
- Alcohol or drug abuse
- Obesity
- Learning difficulties
- Employment problems
- Income problems
- Social isolation
- Childhood abuse
- Severe domestic or marital or legal stress

Fig. 28. Adverse behavioural or psychosocial features associated with the risk of fatal or near-fatal asthma.

Psychotherapeutic interventions such as group or individual family therapy, educational interventions, behavioural therapies, cognitive therapies, cognitive behaviour therapy, relaxation techniques, psychodynamic psychotherapies and counselling, can help with these problems.[125]

Patient education

Successful asthma management involves educating the patient or guardian of an asthmatic child about the disease and its treatment. Education should begin at the time of diagnosis and be a part of every subsequent consultation. Consultations for acute attacks offer an opportunity to discuss and reinforce educational points. Effective educational information will be written, concise and tailored to the individual needs of each patient with age and ability in mind.

First, the patient's preferences and aims for the treatment should be ascertained. The health professional should then ensure the patient has a good understanding of their asthma. The patient should be clear about available treatments and how to use them, and the difference between relief and prevention. Self-management, including how to recognize and deal with an acute exacerbation, should be understood by the patient aided by the development of a personalized asthma

"Successful asthma management involves educating the patient or guardian of an asthmatic child about the disease and its treatment"

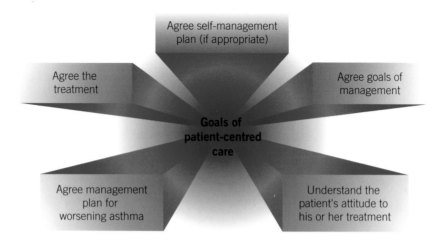

Fig. 29. Goals of patient-centred care.

action plan. Finally, emphasis should be placed on identifying and avoiding the triggers of asthma.

Asthma self-management
Recognizing patients' treatment aims and preferences are key to successful self-management. Figure 29 lists the goals of patient-centred care.

Personalized asthma action plans

Written personalized asthma action plans (PAAPs) improve health outcomes for asthma patients.[126,127] PAAPs are the most effective intervention for routine management, reducing lost days from work and school, hospital admissions, emergency GP consultations, use of reliever medications and for improving lung function. National and international guidelines recommend that written PAAPs are offered to all asthma patients.

> *Patient asthma action plans need to be written, simple and relevant to the individual patient*

PAAPs can be based on peak expiratory flow or symptoms, and can include an emergency course of prednisolone. For most patients under GP care, symptom-based plans with possible supplementary information using peak flows as required are the appropriate course of action. To ensure uptake they need to be written, simple and relevant to the individual. Easy-to-use plans can be obtained from the National Asthma Campaign website at http://www.asthma.org.uk.

To change asthma management behaviour and improve health outcomes a co-ordinated approach of self-management education, regular patient review and a written action plan is likely to be most effective.[128,129]

Acute exacerbations

Acute asthma can result in potentially fatal emergencies. In 1999, 1521 asthma deaths were documented.[2] General practice usually provides front-line emergency care for asthma since most (at least 90%) patients with acute asthma present to primary care.[130,131]

Factors contributing to asthma deaths

Primary care management

An enquiry into asthma deaths by the British Thoracic Association in the early 1980s[132] reported suboptimal delivery of emergency primary care. Inadequate assessment, poor appreciation of exacerbation severity, inadequate emergency treatment and delays in arranging hospital admissions were identified.

More recently two acute asthma audits have revealed an under-use of emergency treatments (such as bronchodilators and oral steroids), suboptimal use of oxygen and self-management plans, and poor availability of peak flow meters and oral steroids in primary care.[130, 131]

Asthma packs (Figure 30) for the surgery or out-of-hours service may encourage optimal treatment by making all acute asthma paraphernalia easily accessible.

Disease severity

The majority of deaths from asthma are associated with a history of severe chronic asthma.[132]

Fig. 30. The acute asthma pack. This should be available in the surgery and the out-of-hours service. Picture and concept courtesy of Dr Hilary Pinnock.

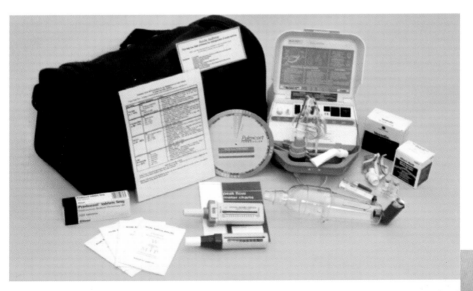

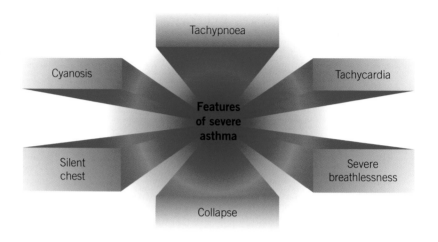

Tachypnoea

Cyanosis

Tachycardia

Features of severe asthma

Silent chest

Severe breathlessness

Collapse

Fig. 31. Clinical features of severe asthma.

Patient psychosocial features

Deaths are associated with adverse behavioural or psychosocial features such as non-compliance with treatment and monitoring, psychiatric illness, denial of asthma, drug abuse or other social problems[14] (see also Psychological and social issues, page 50).

Recognizing acute severe asthma

Most severe attacks develop over a period of between 6 hours or more, the majority over more than 48 hours, allowing time for patients and health care professionals to take effective action. Patients equipped with a written PAAP and a peak flow meter, who have received patient education and have had regular checks of their inhaler technique and treatment compliance, should know how and when to increase their medication and when to seek medical help.

At presentation, the clinical signs and symptoms should be noted and objective clinical measurements taken. The clinical features of acute severe asthma are listed in Figure 31.

Clinical measurements such as PEF or FEV_1 (expressed as the patient's previous best) and pulse oximetry should be taken. Pulse oximetry determines the adequacy of oxygen therapy and the need for arterial blood gas. The aim of oxygen therapy is to maintain $SpO_2 \geq 92\%$.

Proformas are a useful tool for making a systematic initial assessment of asthma severity. Figure 32 lists the BTS/SIGN guidelines[14] for establishing the severity of asthma during an acute exacerbation.

> ❝ *Most severe asthma attacks develop over 6 hours or more, allowing patients and health care professionals time to take effective action* ❞

Severity	Features
Life-threatening asthma*	Any one of the following: •PEF <33% best or predicted •SpO_2 <92% •PaO_2 <8 kPa •Normal $PaCO_2$ (4.6– 6.0 kPa) •Silent chest •Cyanosis •Feeble respiratory effort •Bradycardia •Dysrhythmia •Hypotension •Exhaustion •Confusion •Coma
Acute severe asthma*	•PEF 33–50% best or predicted •Respiratory rate ≥25/min •Heart rate ≥110/min •Inability to complete sentences in 1 breath
Moderate asthma	•Increasing symptoms •PEF 50–75% best or predicted •No features of acute severe asthma
Brittle asthma Type 1	•Wide PEF variability (>40% diurnal variation for >50% of the time over a period of >150 days) despite intense therapy
Type 2	•Sudden severe attacks on a background of apparently well-controlled asthma

*Patients with acute severe or life-threatening asthma should be referred for immediate hospital admission

Fig. 32. Establishing severity of asthma during an acute exacerbation. Based on British Thoracic Society guidelines.[14]

Severity	Features
Life-threatening asthma (PEF <33% best)	• Arrange immediate hospital admission • Give oxygen 40–60% • Give steroids: prednisolone 40–50 mg or IV hydrocortisone 100 mg • Give bronchodilators ideally via nebulizer – either salbutamol 5 mg or terbutaline10 mg – and ipratropium 0.5 mg. (If nebulizer not available give 1 puff ß$_2$-agonist via spacer repeated 10–20 times)
Acute severe asthma (PEF 33–50% best or predicted)	• Consider hospital admission • Give oxygen 40–60% • Give bronchodilators ideally via nebulizer – either salbutamol 5 mg or terbutaline10 mg (if nebulizer not available give 1 puff ß$_2$-agonist via spacer repeated 10–20 times) • Give steroids: prednisolone 40–50mg or IV hydrocortisone 100 mg • If no response to treatment admit
Moderate asthma	• Give bronchodilators ideally via nebulizer – either salbutamol 5 mg or terbutaline10 mg (if nebulizer not available give 1 puff ß$_2$-agonist via spacer repeated 10–20 times) • If PEF 50–75% best/predicted give prednisolone 40–50 mg • Continue or step up normal treatment
Asthma in pregnant patients	• Give immediate oxygen, maintaining saturation over 95% to prevent maternal and foetal hypoxia • Refer immediately those with life-threatening or acute severe asthma • Give drug therapy in same doses as for non-pregnant patients • Admit to hospital if any features of life-threatening or acute severe asthma, or if patient has had a previous near-fatal attack

Fig. 33. Management guidelines for treating adults with acute exacerbations of asthma.[14]

Treatment of acute exacerbations in adults[14]

In the event of an acute attack, oral steroids should be given as quickly as possible (a dose of 40–50 mg prednisolone for adults, 30–40 mg soluble prednisolone for children over 5 years, 20 mg soluble prednisolone for children 2–5 years) and subsequently for at least 5 days or until recovery.

High-dose β_2-agonists via a spacer should also be used as early as possible (10–20 puffs in adults, 10 puffs in children aged 2–5 years with a severe attack or 2–4 puffs in children aged 2–5 years with a moderate exacerbation). Continuous doses of β_2-agonists should be given at 15–30-minute intervals if there is an inadequate response to treatment.

High-flow oxygen should be given to all patients with acute severe asthma (nebulized β_2-agonist should ideally be driven by oxygen, but can be driven by air) unless the patient has COPD, where compressed air would be more appropriate.

The management guidelines[14] for treating adults with acute exacerbations of asthma are listed in Figure 33.

> **During an acute asthma attack, oral steroids should be given as quickly as possible**

When to admit to hospital

Arrange immediate admission for patients with life-threatening asthma, and those with acute severe asthma who do not respond to emergency management. Pregnant patients with acute severe asthma or life-threatening asthma should be referred to hospital immediately.

Consider admitting patients presenting with acute severe asthma, patients who have had previous severe attacks, where attacks are in the afternoon or evening, where patients have had recent nocturnal symptoms or where there is a concern in relation to patients' social circumstances.

In acute asthma in pregnancy, oxygen should be given immediately to maintain oxygen saturation greater than 95% to prevent maternal and foetal hypoxia. Pregnant patients should be referred to hospital *immediately* and drug therapy should be given in the same doses as for non-pregnant patients.

> **Patients with life-threatening asthma, and those with acute severe asthma who do not respond to emergency management, should be referred to hospital immediately**

Follow-up

All acute patients should receive a review within 48 hours of discharge from hospital (or within 48 hours of emergency treatment if not admitted). The health care professional should:
- monitor symptoms and PEF
- check the patient's inhaler technique
- modify treatment according to guidelines for chronic persistent asthma
- provide a written asthma action plan

57

- address potentially preventable contributors to admission.

Since patients with acute asthma present to a variety of health care professionals within or external to the practice (for example, accident and emergency, out-of-hours co-operatives, walk-in centres), it can be difficult to identify recent exacerbations to make adequate follow-up arrangements for the patient. To obtain this information, it may be useful to check regularly the following sources:

- nebulizer use
- computer records
- visit requests
- out-of-hours communications
- A&E notifications
- discharge letters.[130]

"Existing health care models do not maximize the use of GPs' skills"

Structuring respiratory services in primary care

A structured regular review of asthma patients is shown to improve health outcomes regardless of whether the review is undertaken by a GP or a respiratory trained practice nurse.[133,134] British guidelines recommend that all practices keep a list of known asthma patients in order to offer this service, although some patients may not wish to attend review appointments. Presence of a diploma-trained asthma nurse in the practice has been associated with improved outcomes in primary care. Recent research has suggested telephone consultations may be an effective way of following-up those with well controlled asthma.

Good organization is vital to the provision of consistent, high-quality delivery of care. Research has shown that shared care (integration between primary and secondary care) for moderately severe asthma is equally effective as hospital-only care,[135] but it seems the content of delivered care is more important than the setting in which it is given.

"Good organization is vital to the provision of consistent, high-quality delivery of care"

The structure of care is likely to be changed by the Department of Health's intention to introduce 1000 GPs with a special interest (GPwSIs).[136] Existing models do not maximize the use of GPs' skills, so the introduction of GPwSIs might address this by providing greater care specialization to patients and greater peer support to health professionals in the primary care team. Williams et al[137] discuss a potential role for a network of GPwSIs in developing strategies to meet the "primary care governance agenda"[138] and in the improvement of service delivery and cultivation of primary care solutions through three proposed models of service. They highlight a supporting role for GPwSIs in GP re-skilling and promotion of best practice alongside specialist teams.

Auditing care in practice is always a challenge; worthwhile areas in light of the recent British asthma guidelines are listed in Figure 34.

Future developments

Future treatments are likely to target the mechanism of airway remodelling and new therapies such as anti-IgE and phosphodiesterase inhibitors may be the first of many such drugs to evolve as our understanding of asthma pathogenesis increases.[80]

Newer formulations of inhaled steroids which are inactive until lung delivery may be associated with fewer local side-effects.

> *Future treatments are likely to target the mechanism of airway remodelling*

Anti-IgE drugs

Atopic patients respond immunologically to common, naturally occurring allergens by producing IgE antibodies. Anti-IgE drugs are

---

Questions for auditing care in general practice

- Do you have a practice nurse with recognized asthma training/diploma?

- What proportion of patients have clearly recorded justification for an asthma diagnosis in their asthma records? (see http://www.gpiag.org for useful resources)

- What proportion of patients on higher-dose inhaled steroids (>400 mcg BDP or equivalent in children, >800 mcg in adults) have not had a trial of add-on therapy?

- Do you have a system for identifying:
    - children having frequent consultations with respiratory infection?
    - patients with asthma and psychiatric disease or learning disability?
    - those requesting β_2-agonist inhalers frequently (more than one every 6 weeks)?

- How do you identify high-risk patients:
    - patients on Step 3 or more?
    - those having steroid courses for acute asthma/ emergency nebulization/unscheduled appointments for asthma?
    - patients seen in A&E or hospitalized?
    - patients with asthma seeing different doctors?

Fig. 34. British asthma guidelines for auditing care in general practice.

66 *Prevalence of COPD in urban practices is 26%* **99**

designed to treat allergic disease by reducing the concentration of free IgE antibodies in atopic patients irrespective of specific allergens. These drugs may be advantageous in the treatment of multiple allergies, targeting multiple organs (for example lungs, nose and eyes) with convenient dosing (one application every 2 or 4 weeks) that is likely to enhance compliance. Clinical trials have shown that these drugs are associated with a decreased number of exacerbations and use of inhaled corticosteroids in patients with severe persistent allergic asthma.

Phosphodiesterase type 4 inhibitors (roflumilast)

Phosphodiesterase inhibitors that are selective for isoenzyme IV (PDE_4) are distributed differently between tissues and cells thus allowing specific pharmacological intervention. PDE_4 is the predominant isoenzyme in inflammatory cells. Clinical trials report that PDE_4 inhibitors exert potent anti-inflammatory effects on eosinophilic and neutrophilic cells in the airways, resulting in improved lung function in asthma.

CHRONIC OBSTRUCTIVE PULMONARY DISEASE

Definition, epidemiology and aetiology
Definition

66 *COPD is the only common cause of death that is increasing* **99**

Chronic obstructive pulmonary disease (COPD) is a major health care problem. It has a high prevalence, morbidity and mortality, and consequently a high cost.[139–141] The disease consists of inflammation, bronchoconstriction, airflow obstruction and structural changes in the airways, which are irreversible or only partly reversible. A recent definition is:

> "*a disease characterized by airflow limitation that is not fully reversible. The airflow limitation is usually both progressive and associated with an abnormal inflammatory response of the lungs to noxious particles or gases*"[142]

Epidemiology

The facts and figures behind the disease processes collectively known as COPD are bleak. COPD is a progressive chronic condition and is already the third most common cause of death in the UK. By 2020 it is expected to be the third most common cause of death worldwide.[143,144] It is an insidious disease for which genetic, constitutional, familial, behavioural, sociodemographic and environmental factors all predispose patients to its development.[145] Of all the factors implicated, the most important antecedent for the development of COPD is cigarette smoking.[143]

COPD is a major cause of morbidity and mortality. Conservative estimates put morbidity at around 4% in men and 2% in women over age 45.[143] Around 6% of deaths in men and 4% in women, respectively, are attributed to COPD.[143] Morbidity and mortality rates rise sharply after age 50 with prevalence rates ranging from 10% for patients aged 60–75 in semi-rural practices to 26% in urban practices.[146,147] There are approximately 30,000 deaths from COPD annually in the UK, which is around 1 in 20 of all deaths.[148] Furthermore, COPD is the only common cause of death that is increasing.[143]

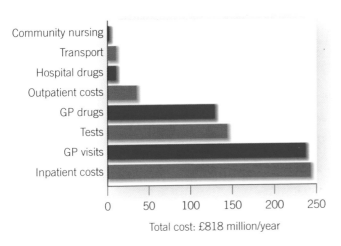

Fig. 35. The cost of managing COPD.

Total cost: £818 million/year

The major burden of COPD is carried by patients and carers[144] and this may be why it is under-resourced. Nevertheless, COPD-related costs in secondary and primary care are high (Figure 35). Patients with COPD are frequent visitors to primary care, often require home visits and account for much of the annual drug budget. In general practice, annual consultation rates for COPD per 10,000 population rise from 417 at age 45–64 to 886 at age 65–74, and 1032 at age 75–84, over four times the rates for angina.[149]

In an average health district, there are around 1000 admissions and 25,000 primary care consultations for COPD per year. According to a British Lung Foundation report, in 1997 the cost implications for the average primary care group were around £540,000 per year.[150] In a primary care trust of 250,000 people, 680 patients will be admitted to hospital with COPD each year and stay on average 10 days.[151] Patients with COPD are more likely than those with asthma to be admitted to hospital and stay on average three times longer. With each hospitalization patients are likely to lose their independence and ability to

❝The major burden of COPD is experienced by the patient and carers❞

cope.[151] A typical primary care trust could expect to experience 54 deaths from COPD each year.[152] Prognosis is worse for severe COPD.

Aetiology

COPD is an umbrella term encompassing chronic bronchitis and emphysema, and patients may have elements of both of these conditions (Figure 36). It is a chronic, slowly progressive disorder characterized predominantly by airways obstruction.[145] There is structural narrowing of the airways that is predominantly irreversible, with a combination of fibrosis, mucus hyperplasia and some alterations in vagal bronchomotor tone.

Chronic bronchitis is caused by hyperplasia of submucosal glands and increased numbers of goblet cells in the epithelium; this leads to mucus hypersecretion. Chronic obstructive bronchitis is associated

Fig. 36. Relationship between chronic bronchitis, asthma and emphysema.

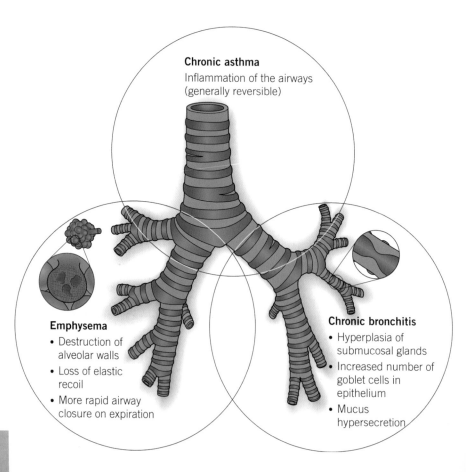

Chronic asthma
Inflammation of the airways
(generally reversible)

Emphysema
- Destruction of alveolar walls
- Loss of elastic recoil
- More rapid airway closure on expiration

Chronic bronchitis
- Hyperplasia of submucosal glands
- Increased number of goblet cells in epithelium
- Mucus hypersecretion

with structural narrowing of the small airways because of chronic inflammation, predominantly through activated T-lymphocytes and macrophages, and this can lead to fibrotic changes.[143] Emphysema is caused by destruction of the alveolar walls, resulting in loss of elastic recoil. This results from parenchymal destruction, with the airways closing more rapidly during expiration. Whether COPD is caused by chronic bronchitis or emphysema, symptoms of breathlessness and discomfort are strongly related to air trapping, which worsens on activity.

Agents causing COPD damage the airways and impair the defence and repair mechanisms within the respiratory system.[153] In addition inflammation increases airway resistance and consequently the thickness of the airway walls, while reducing the driving pressure. Mechanisms implicated in the development of COPD are shown in Figure 37.

Fig. 37. Mechanisms implicated in the development of COPD.

Mechanism	Cause	Implication
Mucus secretion	• Cigarette smoke • Inhaled irritants	• Hyperplasia of submucosal glands • Increased goblet cells • Upregulated mucin genes
Small airways obstruction	• Irritants	• Neutrophil infiltration • Release of chemotactic factors (IL-8, LTB_4) • Secretion of fibrogenic mediators – fibrosis of peripheral airways
Protease–antiprotease imbalance	• Cigarette smoke • Inhaled irritants • Genetic	• Emphysema
Oxidative stress	• Cigarette smoke	• Damage to serum protease inhibitors • Potentiation of elastase activity • Increased mucus secretion • Increased inflammatory response Isoprostane formation
Cellular	• Cigarette smoke	• Inflammation • Increased macrophages • Increased neutrophils
Vascular changes	• Hypoxia	• Pulmonary vasoconstriction Pulmonary hypertension

There is clearly considerable overlap between chronic bronchitis, emphysema and, to a lesser extent, with chronic asthma, and patients with COPD may have a combination of the features of any or all of these disease processes (see Figure 36, page 62).

In advanced disease, levels of arterial oxygen can be low. Chronic hypoxia constricts the walls of the pulmonary arteries; this raises arterial pressure and puts a burden on the heart, often resulting in right-sided heart failure or cor pulmonale. Airway obstruction is largely fixed in COPD, although it can be partially reversed with bronchodilators or other therapy.[145]

> *"Airway obstruction is largely fixed in COPD, although it can be partially reversed with bronchodilators or other therapy"*

Inherited conditions, particularly deficiency of the anti-protease enzyme α_1-antitrypsin, can cause early emphysematous changes in the lungs of relatively young patients whether or not they smoke. Early diagnosis is essential, and a simple blood test can identify family members also at risk. Patients should be encouraged to stop smoking as it significantly increases the risk of rapid lung deterioration.

Diagnosis

Although a thorough history can give a reasonable indication of the diagnosis, spirometry is the gold standard (see Asthma: Diagnosis, page 18).[145,154] A diagnosis of COPD is likely with a history of progressive symptoms; cough, dyspnoea, exacerbations and a smoking history of more than 20-pack years in patients over age 40.[145,154] (One pack-year is the equivalent of smoking 20 cigarettes a day for 1 year.) The higher the number of pack-years, the greater the risk of COPD. Regrettably, patients with mild COPD who would particularly benefit from stopping smoking, rarely attend the practice until it is too late. Symptoms of COPD usually become more evident with age. Lung function naturally declines with age and respiratory damage accumulates. Risk factors for COPD are shown in Figure 38.

> *"Underdiagnosis and under-treatment may be important factors in the high morbidity and mortality from COPD"*

Many patients with COPD could be identified in primary care by targetting:

- smokers with symptoms
- patients on respiratory medication
- patients who attend mainly in the winter months with a "bad chest". These patients are frequently given antibiotics and told to "return if it does not improve".

Underdiagnosis and undertreatment may be important factors in the high morbidity and mortality from COPD.[155] If care is taken during the consultation, rational management can be started early.[154] Early detection and treatment may improve long-term prognosis and prevent irreversible loss of lung function.[155] The presence of co-morbid conditions is a frequent problem. In particular, other smoking-related illnesses, such as heart failure and lung cancer, often co-exist with COPD. It is advisable to refer to a specialist if other disease processes are suspected.[145] (See also "Differential diagnosis", page 98.)

Spirometry

A diagnosis of COPD depends on demonstrating an irreversible component (see also "Asthma: Diagnosis", page 18). Spirometry measures lung function and is the most reliable method for diagnosing COPD.[156] Spirometry can be carried out in general practice, provided a suitable spirometer is available and staff have been properly trained.

Spirometry measures the presence of airflow limitation. The two principal measurements are the forced expiratory volume in 1 second

Who is at risk of developing COPD?
• Smoking history – the higher the number of pack years the greater the risk of COPD (one pack-year being the equivalent of smoking 20 cigarettes/day for 1 year)
• Low birth weight
• Inherited predisposition
• Occupation
• Air pollution including wood smoke and cooking fires in developing countries
• Antiprotease deficiency
• Increasing age
• Gender
• Low socioeconomic status
• Poor diet

Fig. 38. Risk factors for COPD.

(FEV_1) and the forced vital capacity (FVC), which is the total volume of air that can be expelled from the lungs from maximum inhalation to maximum exhalation.

When comparing these two measurements with those predicted for a patient's age, sex, height and ethnicity and looking at the ratio, it is possible to diagnose airflow obstruction. COPD is an obstructive lung disease where FEV_1 is reduced to a greater extent than FVC, which is often referred to as the FEV_1/FVC ratio.[157] A reduction in

Fig. 39. Determining
the severity of COPD.
Taken from BTS
guidelines.[152]

Severity	Signs and symptoms	FEV$_1$ postbronchodilator (% predicted)
Mild	• Smokers cough (occasional or morning) • Little or no breathlessness • No abnormal signs	60–79%
Moderate	• Breathlessness on activity • Cough +/- sputum • Some abnormal signs	40–59%
Severe	• Breathlessness on exertion/rest • Cough and wheeze • Lung hyperinflation • Cyanosis, peripheral oedema and polycythaemia in advanced cases	<40%

FEV$_1$ with relative preservation of FVC indicates and grades airway obstruction. Therefore the FEV$_1$/FVC ratio indicates an obstructive pattern and the FEV$_1$ (post bronchodilator) indicates disease severity.

The ratio of these two measurements, expressed as a percentage, determines the extent of airflow obstruction (see Figure 15, page 22). When the airways are normal, 70–85% of the FVC can be exhaled in the first second. The FEV$_1$ is therefore normally 70–85% of the FVC.

> *The ratio of the FEV$_1$ and the FVC, expressed as a percentage, determines the extent of airflow obstruction*

- A reduced FEV$_1$/FVC ratio indicates airflow obstruction. This could be due to asthma or COPD depending on whether it can be reversed with a bronchodilator.
- A normal FEV$_1$/FVC ratio with a low FEV$_1$ indicates restriction. The patient should generally be referred to a specialist.
- If the FEV$_1$ remains low after a bronchodilator has been given, and the FEV$_1$/FVC ratio is low, COPD is the most likely diagnosis.
- The post-bronchodilator FEV$_1$ on its own indicates disease severity, as shown in Figure 39.

Patients' health needs are related to these categories with both exacerbation rates and the risk of hospitalization rising as the FEV$_1$ falls.

The FVC can vary, so comparing FEV$_1$ with predicted values is a better way of establishing the prognosis. However, both the FVC and the FEV$_1$/FVC ratio can help with differential diagnosis.

A normal FEV_1/FVC ratio rules out a diagnosis of COPD, whereas a normal peak expiratory flow rate (PEFR) does not. A patient with a normal FEV_1 but with symptoms may still be at risk.[158] The post-bronchodilator FEV_1 as a percentage of the predicted FEV_1 is used to classify the severity of COPD.

It is important to test whether any airway obstruction is reversible by carrying out spirometry before and after giving a bronchodilator. If lung function returns to normal or close to normal then the diagnosis is likely to be asthma. If improvement is greater than 400 ml but lung function does not return entirely to normal the patient should be regarded as having mixed disease (ie both COPD and asthma) and treated as such.

High doses of bronchodilator are used to ensure any response can be detected – either 800 mcg salbutamol inhaled via a spacer device or 2.5 mg of nebulized salbutamol. At least two readings before and after administering the bronchodilator must be within 100 ml or 5% of each other.

> **"A normal FEV_1 excludes the diagnosis of COPD whereas a normal PEFR does not"**

How to carry out spirometry

Spirometry should be carried out in patients over 40 with respiratory symptoms (and in those over 35 with signficant symptoms), particularly dyspnoea on activity, cough and wheeze, and a history of smoking.[145] Opportunistic screening, especially case-finding using symptoms such as cough and age as predictors, is a cost-effective way to identify early COPD[159,160] and could help early detection and intervention to prevent further deterioration.[156] Spirometry can also be used for diagnosing or monitoring occupational lung disease.

Patients should be asked to avoid:
- smoking 24 hours before the test
- alcohol 4 hours before the test
- eating a large meal 2 hours before the test
- taking a short-acting bronchodilator 4 hours before the test
- taking long-acting bronchodilators 24 hours before the test
- vigorous exercise 30 minutes before the test
- wearing restrictive clothing.

> **"Opportunistic screening, especially case-finding using cough and age as predictors, is a cost-effective way to identify early COPD"**

Spirometry should always be performed by someone adequately trained in undertaking the procedure. Before interpreting the results the British Thoracic Society suggests the following criteria should be satisfied:
- there are at least three technically satisfactory readings
- the expiratory volume/time traces are smooth, convex upwards, and free from irregularities that suggest either variable submaximal effort or coughing

	Obstructive	Restrictive	Combined
	FEV_1 low	FEV_1 low	FEV_1 low
	FVC low	FVC low	FVC low
	FEV_1/FVC ratio normal/low	FEV_1/FVC ratio normal/high	FEV_1/FVC ratio low

Fig. 40. Using spirometry results to determine whether a patient has obstruction, restriction or both.

- there are at least two readings of FEV_1 that are within 100 ml or 5% of the other
- the recording has been continued long enough for a volume plateau to be reached on the volume–time plot. This can take up to 15 seconds in patients with severe COPD.

Abbreviated efforts will underestimate FVC. The best FEV_1 and best FVC values should be recorded.

Explain the purpose of the examination and the need for extra effort from the patient to get maximal results. Instructions such as "I want to measure how hard and fast you can breath" are helpful and may be sufficient.

Explain the procedure in simple language and demonstrate a deep inspiration, proper placement of the mouthpiece, and blasting of air into the tube. Blow for at least four seconds to make the demonstration as realistic as possible.

Ask the patient to loosen any tight clothing and remove dentures (if they are not secure). Install a new mouthpiece into the spirometer hose. Ask the patient to sit during the examination. Ask the patient to raise their chin and extend their neck slightly. A noseclip may be placed on their nose. Clips may be removed between trials. Get the patient to blow into the spirometer until they have completely emptied their lungs. The following instructions may be helpful:

- "Take a great big deep breath of air as far as you can inhale." (The examinee should inhale from room air).
- "Put the mouthpiece into your mouth and seal your lips tightly around it." (Demonstrate the correct technique)
- "Blast your air into the tube as hard and fast as you can." (The exhalation should be made with the lips tight around the mouthpiece with maximal force and speed)
- "Keep on blowing out the same breath of air, until I tell you to stop."

Review the procedure and correct any problems from the trial. Repeat for a minimum of three blows or until adeqaute quality has been achieved.

66 Spirometry should always be performed by someone adequately trained in undertaking the procedure 99

Lung function is insufficient on its own for assessing response to any therapeutic intervention. Assessments of exercise tolerance, functional status, and quality of life should also be considered.[160,161] Figure 40 illustrates how to interpret spirometry data in terms of obstruction and restriction.

Interpreting reversibility with spirometry results

Many patients demonstrate some reversibility, but the result is only clinically relevant if the FEV_1 rises by at least 400 ml. Patients with this degree of reversibility are likely to have an asthmatic component to their disease, will be more likely to respond to asthma therapies and have a better prognosis.

Substantial reversibility (≥400 ml) suggests the patient has asthma, and if lung function returns to normal this indicates asthma alone. However, if the FEV_1 does not return to normal, but there is a rise of 400 ml, it is reasonable to describe these patients as having "mixed disease" – a combination of COPD and asthma.

If the FEV_1 rises to over 80% of normal these patients have asthma. Patients with limited reversibility 200 ml (15%) or under are recognized as having COPD. (See also "Differential diagnosis", page 98.)

66 The result is only significant if the FEV_1 rises by at least 400 ml 99

Smoking cessation

Smoking is the most preventable cause of premature death and disability in the developed world. One in four smokers will develop COPD and the risk is higher the greater the total tobacco exposure.[162] Smoking cessation is of substantial benefit to lung function,[163] effectively slowing the decline in FEV_1 seen in smokers. The effects of smoking on lung function are shown in Figure 41.

Fig. 41. The effects of smoking on declining lung function.
Reproduced from BMJ 1977;1:1645–648 with permission from the BMJ Publishing Group.

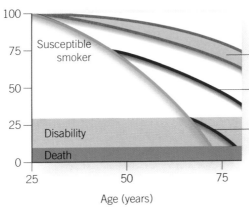

Lung function FEV$_1$ (percentage of value at age 25)

Susceptible smoker

Never smoked or not susceptible to smoke

Stopped smoking at 45 years

Stopped smoking at 65 years

Disability

Death

Age (years)

Time after last cigarette	Benefit
20 minutes	• Blood pressure and pulse return to normal • Circulation improves in feet and hands, making them warmer
8 hours	• Oxygen levels in the blood return to normal • Chances of a heart attack start to fall
24 hours	• Carbon monoxide is eliminated from the body • Mucus and other debris start to clear from the lungs
48 hours	• Nicotine is no longer detectable in the body • Ability to taste and smell improves
72 hours	• Breathing becomes easier as the bronchial tubes relax • Energy levels increase
2–12 weeks	• Circulation improves in the body so walking is easier
3–9 months	• Breathing problems such as cough, shortness of breath and wheeze show improvement with lung function increasing by about 5–10%
5 years	• Risk of heart attack falls to about half of that of a smoker
10 years	• Risk of lung cancer falls to half that of a smoker • Risk of heart attack similar to someone who has never smoked

Fig. 42. Benefits of giving up smoking habit shown in terms of time after last cigarette. Patients are unlikely to consider stopping unless they can perceive a tangible benefit.

Smoking cessation should be the first step for patients with mild airway obstruction.[164] Smokers with early COPD who were assigned to a smoking-cessation programme had fewer respiratory symptoms (chronic cough, chronic phlegm production, wheezing and shortness of breath) after 5 years of follow-up.[165]

Some smokers, especially those who have smoked for many years, may be reluctant to stop, as they believe the damage is irreversible. Patients are unlikely to consider stopping unless they can identify a tangible benefit. Once lung function has deteriorated it cannot be restored, but the *rate* of deterioration can be reduced. It is never too late to stop and the benefits start immediately (Figure 42).

Giving anti-smoking advice

Guidelines[142, 145] recommend practitioners discuss smoking routinely in every consultation. However, health professionals and patients often prefer to link smoking advice to smoking-related problems. Indeed, some patients are unhappy about receiving advice before they are ready to give up.

Brief smoking cessation advice given by GPs has been shown to be simple and effective.[166,167] For every 40 patients given brief advice (where smokers are systematically identified and offered advice routinely) there will be one extra quitter (NNT 40).[166,167] Looked at another way, for every 40 smokers seen in consultation who are not offered advice, one smoker who might otherwise have given up may continue to smoke. So every consultation is an opportunity to make an impact, and continued or follow-up advice can assist sustained abstinence.[167] However, this should be viewed as a bare minimum as attempts at quitting without adequate support are much more likely to fail than those where pharmacological and psychological support is provided. Failed attempts are associated with a refractory period in which smokers will not attempt further smoking cessation. A summary of the ways a GP can help smokers to quit is shown in Figure 43.

As smoking-related COPD is preventable, one approach to reducing the associated morbidity and mortality could be for practices to target all smokers among their patients. However, while this would prevent disease in its early stages, the approach is not very practical.

More intensive individual counselling by an experienced therapist (in association with pharmacotherapy) outside the primary care setting may help motivated quitters.[168]

Nicotine replacement therapy

In 1998, the Department of Health in the UK published a report by an expert panel on smoking cessation and nicotine replacement

66 Smoking is the most preventable cause of death in the UK 99

66 Some patients are unhappy about receiving smoking cessation advice before they are ready to give up 99

therapy (NRT).[169] The report stated that tobacco addiction should be taken as seriously as other drug or alcohol addictions, and that NRT should be available on prescription. This is especially important in the lower-income groups, where the effects of smoking appear to cause the highest rates of morbidity and mortality, and who are least likely to consider smoking cessation or the benefits of NRT.[169]

> *Nicotine replacement therapy should be directed at smokers who are motivated to quit*

Although not a magical cure, NRT increases the chances of success and over 80 research articles have reported a proven efficacy.[167] NRT minimizes many of the physiological and psychomotor withdrawal symptoms frequently experienced after stopping smoking, it may increase the likelihood that a person remains abstinent and can be used as part of a smoking cessation strategy.[170] It gives smokers the chance to break their nicotine addiction by gradually reducing the amount of nicotine in the body. NRT is available as:

- gum
- transdermal patches
- nasal spray
- inhalator
- sublingual tablets.

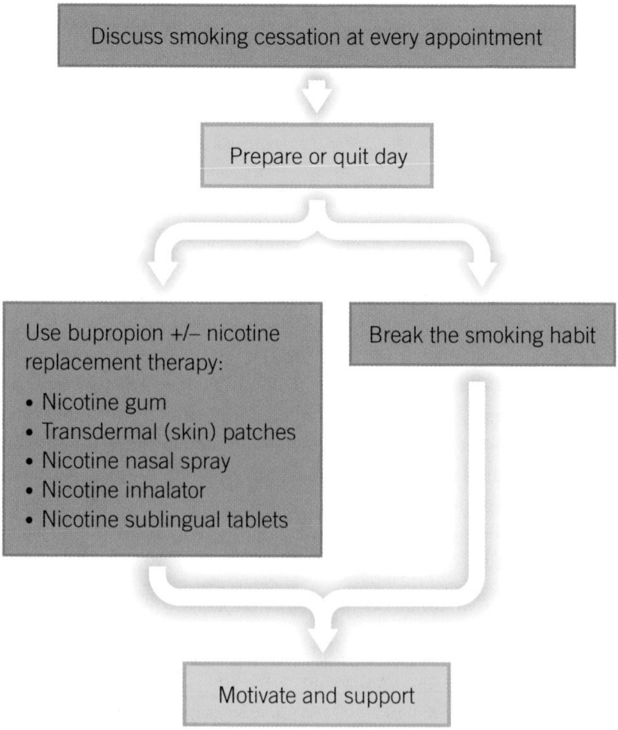

Fig. 43. How GPs can help smokers to quit.

Discuss smoking cessation at every appointment

Prepare or quit day

Use bupropion +/– nicotine replacement therapy:

- Nicotine gum
- Transdermal (skin) patches
- Nicotine nasal spray
- Nicotine inhalator
- Nicotine sublingual tablets

Break the smoking habit

Motivate and support

All NRT products must be used in sufficient quantity for sufficient time. All the commercially available forms are effective as part of a strategy to promote smoking cessation and have a very benign side-effect profile. They increase long term-quit rates approximately 1.5- to 2-fold regardless of setting.[167]

Use of NRT should be directed preferentially to smokers who are motivated to quit (demonstrated by their request for help) and have high levels of nicotine dependency. This may be assessed by asking the patient how soon they have a cigarette after waking and how many they smoke each day. Smokers who have a cigarette within 30 minutes of getting up are highly addicted and will need higher strengths of NRT.

Choice of therapy should reflect patient need, tolerability, and cost. Patches are likely to be easier to use than gum or nasal spray in the primary care setting. There is minimal evidence that giving a repeated course of NRT to patients who have relapsed after recently using nicotine patches will result in a small additional probability of quitting.[167]

Gum

Chewing the gum releases nicotine, which is absorbed through the mouth lining. It comes in a 2 mg and 4 mg dose and can be flavoured. Patients are advised to use a piece of gum when they would be having a cigarette for up to 3 months and then to gradually reduce this.

The gum should be chewed slowly to allow the nicotine to be released and 2 mg should be used as the starting dose. Some smokers complain about the taste, but it improves with use. For highly dependent smokers, or those who have no success with 2 mg gum, 4 mg gum should be offered. A prediction of this is time to first cigarette in the morning. If less than 30 minutes this suggests greater addiction and a higher strength is probably needed.

Nicotine gum can be of limited use in some smokers. Absorption may be impaired when the gum is taken with coffee or acidic drinks, and oral and gastric side-effects can be a problem.[171] Transferring the dependency from cigarettes to the gum[170] may result in addiction in some patients. Adequate dosing is important, but gum can be offered on a fixed dose or on an *ad lib* basis.[172]

Other types of NRT (patches, nasal spray, inhalator and tablets) aim to avoid some of the problems associated with nicotine gum.[167] All five forms are significantly more effective than placebo (or no NRT) in helping smokers abstain.[167]

Skin patches

Transdermal skin patches release nicotine slowly over 16 or 24 hours, maintaining a steady level in the body, and resulting in plasma levels

> **❝Nicotine replacement therapy increases the chances of success of smokers quitting their habit❞**

73

similar to the trough levels seen in heavy smokers.[173] The patches come in various doses between 7 mg and 22 mg. Smokers are advised to use the highest doses available at first, cutting down gradually. This method is successful in smokers who consume over 15 cigarettes a day. Moreover, 8 weeks of patch therapy is equally effective as longer courses, and there is no evidence that tapered therapy is better than abrupt withdrawal.

Wearing the patch only during waking hours (16 hours a day) is as effective as wearing it for 24 hours a day.[166] There is borderline evidence that there is a small benefit from use of the nicotine patch at higher doses than the standard-dose patch. These may be considered for heavy smokers (≥30 a day) or for patients relapsing because of persistent craving and withdrawal symptoms on standard-dose therapy.[167]

> **"Transdermal patches appear successful in smokers who consume over 15 cigarettes/day."**

Nasal spray

The Nicorette nasal spray contains a small bottle of nicotine solution that is sprayed into the nasal passages and is used when there is an urge for a cigarette. Rapid absorption of the nicotine into the nasal mucosa replicates the way a smoker experiences nicotine absorption from a cigarette; so this method may be useful for heavily addicted patients. The nasal spray is available only on private prescription and, although effective, can have an irritant effect on the nasal mucosa.

Nicorette inhalator

The Nicorette inhalator consists of a plastic mouthpiece and a container for a nicotine cartridge. The smoker sucks on the inhalator as they would a cigarette. For some people it is an effective way of replacing the hand-to-mouth action that has become a habit. The nicotine is absorbed in the mouth and throat and does not pass into the lungs.

The cost of these therapies is roughly similar and about the same as smoking cigarettes if they are bought without a prescription.

> **"The Nicorette inhalator is a very effective way of replacing the smoker's hand to mouth action"**

Nicotine tablets

Sublingual nicotine tablets are dissolved under the tongue when cravings occur and can be useful for those heavily addicted to nicotine. The most common side-effects are nausea, dyspepsia and hiccup, which are nicotine-related. As with gum, research suggests that an adequate dose with a regular schedule of administration is clinically important.[174,175]

Combination therapy

There is some evidence of a small benefit from combining the nicotine patch with *ad-lib* dosing of another form of NRT such as the inhalator or sublingual lozenges.[167] Combination therapy may be considered for patients unable to quit using a single type of NRT or with heavily addicted patients.[167]

There is no evidence that one form of NRT is better than any other. Clearly none of these products alone offers a magical "cure" for the smoking habit.

Support or counselling, although beneficial in increasing the likelihood of quitting, is not essential because the effectiveness of NRT is largely independent of any additional support[167] (Figure 44).

Antidepressant therapy

Although NRT is the most widely used pharmacotherapy for smoking cessation, some people prefer a treatment that is not nicotine based. Patient preferences, side-effect profiles, cost and availability need to be considered before a choice is made.

The observations that a history of depression is found more frequently among smokers than non-smokers, that cessation may

Intervention	Quit rate after 6 months
Brief advice from a health care professional (3–10 minutes)	2–3%
Advice and NRT	6%
Advice, NRT and ongoing support	8–25%

Fig. 44. Success rates for quitting smoking compared with no intervention.

precipitate depression, and that nicotine may have antidepressant effects provide a rationale for prescribing antidepressants for smoking cessation.[171] Two drugs used to treat depression – bupropion and nortriptyline – are useful for some smokers who are trying to quit.[176]

Bupropion (Zyban) is essentially an antidepressant used in the USA that has been found to reduce the effects of withdrawal symptoms and the desire to smoke by sensitizing the brain's nicotine receptors.[177] Bupropion is normally prescribed for 2 months at a dose of 300 mg/day. The smoker is usually committed to stopping smoking on the eighth day of the course and requires regular follow-up and support.

In smoking cessation trials, bupropion more than doubled cessation rates. It can also be helpful in those who do not find nicotine replacement useful.

Bupropion has some side-effects; the most important is the risk of seizure. At the dose for smoking cessation the risk is estimated to be 1

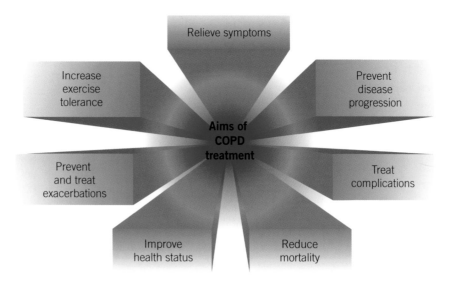

Fig. 45. Aims of
treatment for COPD.

in 1000, so it should not be given to those with a history of seizure.[176] Other contraindications are a history of bulimia, anorexia, hepatic cirrhosis, bipolar disorder or those on monoamine oxidase inhibitors.

Trials of the tricyclic antidepressant nortriptyline suggest this also doubles quit rates. Side-effects include nausea and sedation; it may also cause urinary retention and can be dangerous in overdose.[175] Smokers with a history of depression or mild current depression have not been shown to fare better with antidepressants than with NRT. Patient preferences, cost, availability and side-effects must be taken into account.

Nortriptyline may be considered a second-line therapy as it has more side-effects. All the treatments can produce clinically significant adverse effects; however, regardless of the clinical side-effects associated with both antidepressant drugs, less than 10% of patients typically stop taking the medication because of any adverse effect.[176]

Treatment of stable COPD

Although FEV_1 is an important measurement in COPD, the need for treatment is difficult to assess by measuring lung function alone. By virtue of the definition of the disease there is limited scope for improvement, and also the disease is chronic and progressive deterioration is inevitable. For the patient, symptoms, health status, exercise capacity and reduced frequency of exacerbations may be more important than objective lung measurements.[179]

Patients may not see exacerbations as the most problematic aspect of their disease; their concerns centre around access to healthcare, understanding medical decisions and overall wellbeing.

Patients also perceive their symptoms differently. A patient with very limited lung function may not complain of breathlessness, while someone with essentially good lung function may perceive their symptoms to be extremely disabling and life-limiting. Clinical objectivity is therefore not easy. The aims of treatment are shown in Figure 45.

Medication
The aim of medical treatment of COPD is to achieve maximal airway function through regular use of bronchodilators at the maximum tolerated levels.[142,145] Although no medication will change the natural history of the disease, it may relieve symptoms, improve health status or quality of life and reduce exacerbation rates and risk of hospitalization.

Many drug treatments used for asthma are also used for COPD, although there are clearly different indications and recommendations for use. Patients with COPD will not respond to treatments in the same way as patients with asthma because the disease process is different. Recommendations for treatment of COPD based on the GOLD guidelines[158] are shown in Figure 46.

Bronchodilators
Bronchodilators are the mainstay of pharmacological treatment for COPD. They are thought to decrease dyspnoea and improve breathing by deflating the lung and reducing residual volume (reduce air trapping).[180] ß$_2$-agonists, anticholinergics and theophylline are effective bronchodilators; the choice depends on the individual's response to treatment.

Bronchodilators are believed to work by relaxing smooth muscle in the airways, or preventing constriction of the airways, increasing their diameter. In many patients combining ß$_2$-agonists and anticholinergics may provide additional benefit and should be considered when one alone produces an inadequate response.

Short-acting ß$_2$-agonists (salbutamol, terbutaline)
Short-acting ß$_2$-agonists (SABAs) help relieve the symptoms of COPD. They work predominantly by relaxing the airway smooth muscle, although several additional effects on the airway may contribute to their therapeutic effects. These drugs can be used regularly or as required for COPD, although the benefit:risk ratio suggests that daily dose should not exceed 1 mg.[148]

This is very different from their use in treating asthma, where the medication is considered efficacious only when used as sparingly as possible, and preferably used as needed, in all but those with severe disease. In COPD, SABAs can increase FEV_1, reduce breathlessness, increase exercise capacity and improve health.[181]

> **"**Patients with COPD will not respond to treatments in the same way as patients with asthma because the disease process is different**"**

77

The side-effects of ß₂-agonists are palpitations and tremor, so care must be taken in elderly patients with a known cardiac history. Potassium levels may also fall with regular use, and this should be checked at least twice-yearly.

> *Bronchodilators are the mainstay of pharmacological treatment for COPD*

Long-acting ß₂-agonists (formoterol, salmeterol)

The long-acting ß₂-agonists (LABAs) formoterol (Foradil, Oxis) and salmeterol (Serevent) work in a similar way to SABAs but have a longer duration of action, lasting around 12 hours. Studies have shown

Stage	Recommended treatment
0 At risk	• Avoidance of risk factors • Influenza vaccination
I Mild COPD	• Add short-acting bronchodilator when needed
II Moderate COPD	• Add regular treatment with one or more long-acting bronchodilators (anticholinergic or β-agonist) • Add rehabilitation
III Severe COPD	• Add inhaled glucocorticosteroids if repeated exacerbations
IV Very severe COPD	• Add long-term oxygen if there is chronic respiratory failure • Consider surgical referral

Fig. 46. Recommendations for treating COPD based on the GOLD guidelines.[164]

that in COPD, LABAs can increase FEV_1, increase exercise tolerance, improve health status and improve night-time symptoms.[148,182,183]

Also, LABAs may reduce infective exacerbations. This may be due to an increase in the body's defence mechanisms or it may be that as baseline breathlessness is reduced, exacerbations are less easy to recognize.[148] Guidelines recommend that LABAs are considered for moderately severe COPD or in those with mild disease with respect to lung function, lifestyle limitation or persistent symptoms despite using SABAs.

Anticholinergics (ipratropium bromide)

Anticholinergics are at least as effective as ß₂-agonists for treating COPD, unlike for asthma.[143] In addition to the bronchodilation, which is caused by a reduction in vagal cholinergic tone, anticholinergics may also reduce hypersecretion of mucus.

The side-effects mainly result from their topical action, since little is absorbed systemically. Side-effects include dry mouth, urinary retention, constipation, bitter taste and glaucoma. To reduce the risk of glaucoma, patients using a nebulized anticholinergic should use a mouthpiece instead of a mask.

Anticholinergics have a greater and more prolonged bronchodilator effect in COPD than asthma, and use with a $ß_2$-agonist may increase bronchodilation.[143]

Long-acting anticholinergics (tiotropium)

Although ipratropium is an effective drug its duration is 4 to 6 hours. Long-acting anticholinergics are more recent additions to the therapeutic field. Tiotropium bromide is structurally related to ipratropium bromide but it has a unique property of kinetic selectivity and very long duration of action of more than 24 hours. Tiotropium is suitable for once-daily inhalation in COPD, and early research suggests that it offers more sustained bronchodilation, improved dyspnoea, health-related quality of life, and exacerbations than four times daily treatment with ipratropium bromide.[188, 189] A recent study showed at least comparable improvements in dyspnoea, health-related quality of life, and exacerbations when compared with twice daily 50 mcg salmeterol .[184]

Long-acting anticholinergics have been shown to relieve dyspnoea and improve exercise tolerance, which are the most frequent complaints of COPD patients.[185,186]

Oral ß₂-agonists

Ideally, oral $ß_2$-agonists should only be considered in patients with COPD who have difficulty using an inhaler or will not consider using one. Systemic side-effects are likely with oral preparations.

Methylxanthines

Methylxanthines, such as theophylline, are usually reserved for more severe disease because of their narrow therapeutic range and the risk of side-effects. Theophylline is also indicated as an additional bronchodilator in patients not controlled on regular anticholinergic therapy. The therapeutic effect and side-effects are related to plasma concentration, plasma levels should be between 10 and 20 mg/l. Side-effects include nausea and vomiting, headache, restlessness, gastro-oesophageal reflux, diuresis, cardiac arrhythmias (plasma concentration >20 mg/l) and epileptic seizures (with a plasma concentration usually >30 mg/l).

To reduce the risk of side-effects, the drug should be introduced slowly and the plasma levels must be kept below 20 mg/l. Many factors can affect the plasma level such as smoking, other drugs (rifampicin, cimetidine, erythromycin, ciprofloxacin), congestive heart failure and liver disease. Regular blood monitoring is required.

❝Long-acting anticholinergics have been shown to relieve dyspnoea, which is the most frequent complaint of COPD patients ❞

Phosphodiesterase type 4 inhibitors (roflumilast, cilomilast)

While methylxanthines have important clinical benefits in patients with COPD, they are limited by side-effects. In one recent study there was a 39% dropout. Much of the clinical benefit is thought to be from PDE_4 inhibition with side-effects due to other actions. As a result, selective PDE_4 inhibitors have been developed that have most of the clinical advantages but far fewer side-effects.

Studies suggest this drug class has a broad range of important anti-inflammatory effects. Initial trials have shown improved lung function and health-related quality of life, and a trend towards reduced exacerbations. Side-effects were substantially less than for methylxanthines, with 3-4% suffering from headache, abdominal pain, nausea and diarrhoea. This appears to be an exciting therapy for the future.

> *Long-acting anticholinergics have been shown to relieve dyspnoea, which is the most frequent complaint of COPD patients*

Inhaled corticosteroids (budesonide, fluticasone)

The inflammation associated with COPD does not appear to be suppressed by inhaled or oral corticosteroids, even at high doses. Therefore patients highly responsive to ICS probably have concomitant asthma.[187] Research suggests that corticosteroids reduce exacerbations in COPD and may reduce decline in pulmonary function.[188–190, 256] They should therefore be considered for patients who experience frequent exacerbations, and whose lung function is less than 50% predicted.[142,145, 261] It is important to consider side-effects and cost .[142,145]

Combination therapy for COPD

Recent guidelines from the UK National Institute for Clinical Excellence state that there is good supportive evidence for combinations of:[261]

- ß-agonist and anticholinergic
- ß-agonist and theophylline
- anticholinergic and theophylline
- ß-agonist and inhaled corticosteroid.

NICE recommends that combining therapies from different classes is likely to increase clinical benefit and have fewer side-effects than increasing individual drug dosages. Two of these combinations are also available in single inhalers.

> *Corticosteroids are widely used in COPD but their role remains unclear*

1. ß-agonists and anticholinergics

Guidelines advocate that for moderate and severe COPD, combination therapies with $ß_2$-agonists and anticholinergics should be considered.[142,145] Combination therapy may produce greater symptom relief with fewer side-effects than increasing the dose of single agents, and may be more convenient for patients, although in some instances more expensive to prescribe.[190]

2. ICS and LABAs (Seretide, Symbicort)

Based on the evidence of effectiveness of LABAs and ICS in more severe COPD, studies have been conducted with higher-dose combination formulations. These have shown significant improvements in quality of life, symptoms, need for relief bronchodilators and reductions in exacerbations. Guidelines recommend their use in patients for whom the individual components would be recommended.[257, 258]

Mucolytics (carbocisteine, mecysteine hydrochloride)

Because chronic bronchitis is associated with hypersecretion of mucus, mucolytics may be considered for treatment. Their effectiveness in COPD is, however, still debated.[143,191,192] There is little evidence of an improvement in lung function with mucolytics.[143]

Anti-oxidants

N-acetyl cysteine has been shown in recent studies to reduce exacerbations of COPD. The role of this class of therapy has recently been re-evaluated and recommended for consideration in patients with a chronic productive cough.[261]

Vaccinations

In selected patients with recurrent exacerbations of non-viral bronchitis, vaccination against *Haemophilus influenzae* may reduce the number and severity of bronchitis episodes over the winter months.[193] Although there are no specific studies in COPD, vaccination of patients with chronic respiratory disease against influenza has been shown to reduce hospital attendance, admission rates and death rates for influenza.[194,195] Vaccinating patients against *Pneumococcus spp.* also reduces incidence of invasive pneumococcal strains and is cost-effective.[196]

Antibiotics

A meta-analysis of controlled trials of antibiotic therapy showed a statistically significant, but small, benefit of antibiotics in terms of clinical outcome and lung function in COPD.[197] There is no evidence that antibiotics are effective for preventing exacerbations, and they are not useful for non-infective exacerbations, so prophylactic use is unnecessary.

The choice of antibiotic should be based on the likely sensitivity of the organism. The antibiotic should be changed if sensitivity results are available or if a viral infection is later found to be the cause.[198]

Treatment should be for 10–14 days and stopped if the patient has responded.[143] If there is no response, a different broad-spectrum antibiotic may be tried.

> *In selected patients vaccination against Haemophilus influenzae may reduce the number and severity of bronchitis episodes over the winter months*

> *A meta-analysis of controlled trials of antibiotics showed a statistically significant, but small, benefit of antibiotics in terms of clinical outcome and lung function in COPD*

Medication devices

Metered-dose inhalers (MDIs) are recommended for most COPD patients.[142–145] They are the cheapest delivery devices but may need a spacer to increase drug deposition and encourage appropriate use. All patients should have their inhaler technique assessed to determine which device is the most suitable. There are no adequately powered studies comparing inhaler device efficacy in non-acute COPD.[199]

66 All patients considered for a home nebulizer should have a formal assessment by a respiratory physician 99

Nebulizer assessment

The benefit of nebulized therapy in COPD is unclear and unproven. Most patients can be treated with MDIs and spacers or dry powder devices;[200–203] a few, however, may benefit from higher doses of medication, in which case nebulizer assessment may be appropriate.[204,205] Patients may also gain some benefit from the moistening or cooling effects of the aerosol generated by a nebulizer.[148]

All patients considered for a home nebulizer should be formally assessed by a respiratory physician.[205] This will ensure the correct diagnosis is established, the device is used optimally, the response to the nebulizer home trial is determined, and lung function measurements are taken.[115]

The BTS guidelines produced in 1997 give guidance on nebulizer assessment and use.[115] Clearly, nebulized therapies are significantly more expensive and patients are more likely to experience side-effects, but they are easy to administer with a compressor. The compressors need to be cleaned and maintained regularly for optimal use and serviced annually.[152] In terms of efficacy and cost-effectiveness, nebulized therapies should be reserved for patients with the most severe airflow obstruction when other forms of inhaler have failed and where benefit has been demonstrated.[201]

66 LTOT lessens polycythaemia, reduces progression of pulmonary hypertension, improves long-term survival, improves sleep quality, reduces cardiac arrhythmias, and increases renal blood flow 99

Patients often have great faith in compressors and nebulizers, and it is difficult to be objective because patients may feel they gain significant symptomatic benefit from nebulized compared with inhaled therapy without any significant changes in lung function.

Oxygen therapy

Patients with chronic lung disease develop chronic hypoxaemia that is related to the progression of their underlying condition. Over the last 20 years, domiciliary oxygen therapy has become a major form of treatment for hypoxaemic patients with COPD. Domiciliary oxygen services will supply oxygen to the patient's home, advise on its use, regularly service equipment and provide 24-hour call-out.

Two definitive studies on long-term oxygen therapy (LTOT) reported improved survival in patients with hypoxic chronic lung disease.[205,206] In England and Wales, oxygen requirements are assessed in secondary care and prescribed in primary care. In Scotland, oxygen requirements are both assessed and prescribed by chest physicians.[207]

There are clear criteria for referral for LTOT. Patients should:

- be stable
- have a resting PaO_2 of 7.3 kPa or SaO_2 at or below 88% with or without hypercapnia, or between 7.3 and 8.0 kPa or an SaO_2 of 89%
- have evidence of polycythaemia, haematocrit >55%, nocturnal hypoxia, peripheral oedema or pulmonary hypertension.

Moreover, specialist assessment is required and any oxygen prescription should include the source, method of delivery and duration of use.[208]

LTOT lessens polycythaemia, reduces progression of pulmonary hypertension, improves long-term survival, improves sleep quality, reduces cardiac arrhythmias, and increases renal blood flow.[206, 207] Trials of LTOT showed the benefits of using oxygen for 19 hours/day was the most effective for disease survival.[206, 207] This was followed by use for 15 hours, with usage for 12 hours showing only very marginal effect on the disease. [206, 207]

LTOT appears to improve survival in a selected group of COPD patients with severe hypoxaemia. It appears to be less effective in those with moderate hypoxaemia or nocturnal oxygen desaturation alone.[209] But despite the benefits, the restriction to independence and the reinforcement of chronic illness may make compliance difficult.

LTOT is usually delivered via an oxygen concentrator (Figure 47). This is backed up by an oxygen cylinder and portable oxygen (Figure 48) to encourage independence.

"Oxygen concentrators are the usual method of delivery of LTOT"

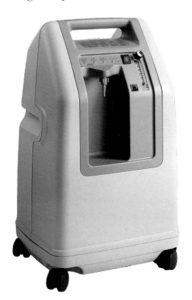

Fig. 47. An oxygen concentrator.

An adequate length of oxygen tubing should be provided to help the patient move around the house. Nasal cannulae are commonly used for low flow rates as they are more comfortable and allow eating and talking. Humidification is not necessary at low flow rates.[148] Compliance with LTOT is extremely variable and difficult to assess, as patients will often overestimate the time spent on the machine. The providers of the concentrators can monitor actual use and inform the GP if use is inadequate to merit a cylinder instead of a concentrator.

Prescribing portable cylinders may encourage patients to remain mobile. The PD, DD and PA2 cylinders are available on prescription, but the carrying cases have to be bought separately. The PD is the heaviest and provides 150 minutes of gas when the flow rate is set at 2 l/min.

Fig. 48. Portable oxygen encourages independence.

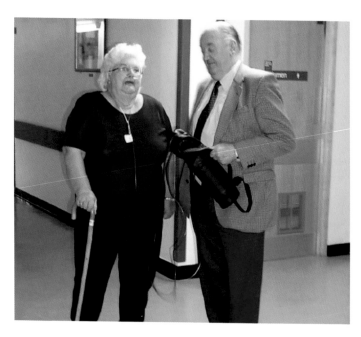

It can also give variable flow rates from 0.5–15 l/min. The DD and PA2 are lighter and provide about 230 minutes of gas when set at 2 l/min. The cylinder heads are integral so patients do not have to change them, which can be a problem for patients with limited manual dexterity.

Liquid oxygen is provided from a base unit in the patient's home. A small portable unit can be refilled from this. Liquid oxygen is not available on prescription in the UK.[208] Patients can buy it privately, although this option is expensive.[209]

There are several considerations to make when choosing an oxygen system for a patient. The method of gas production, weight, size, cost, ease of refilling and maintenance, availability and portability should all be taken into account. The advantage of liquid oxygen reservoirs are that they last 5 to 7 days (at 2 l/min) and can be used to refill portable units.

Some patients equate breathlessness with low oxygen levels. These patients may put pressure on their GP to provide oxygen unnecessarily. Prescribing oxygen for such patients may in fact serve only to reinforce an image of negative chronic illness. *Ad hoc* prescription of oxygen for symptomatic relief of breathlessness provides subjective but scientifically unproven benefit. There is a small group of patients in the palliative stages of the disease that may gain psychological benefit from oxygen provision and in these instances, oxygen provision is appropriate even if normal selection criteria are not met. However, they will require evaluation for possible carbon dioxide retention. Figure 49 illustrates the assessment of oxygen need in COPD.

> *"Liquid oxygen is not currently available on prescription and is provided from a base unit in the patient's home from which a small portable unit can be refilled"*

Mask or nasal prongs?

While some patients prefer a mask, not all can tolerate one. For low oxygen flow rates, nasal prongs are convenient, simple to use and usually more comfortable and less claustrophobic for the wearer. Nasal prongs allow patients to talk and eat during oxygen therapy and can be used at the same time as nebulized medication. Even mouth breathers can benefit from nasal prongs, although the inspired oxygen may be lower than normally expected. To prevent the nasal passages becoming dry, patients can use a water-soluble lubricant. Patients should be advised to drink plenty of liquid as oxygen can dry the mucous membranes and also make pulmonary secretions thicker so they are less easy to expectorate. Whether using a mask or nasal prongs, putting gauze or disposable foam wraps on the tubing may stop sores developing.

Oxygen cylinders are one of the largest medical expenses in primary care. High use in individual patients merits a thorough review.

Exacerbations

COPD is not a stable disease and patients experience periodic worsening of symptoms or exacerbations. Patients with a definite diagnosis and who respond to treatment, do not require further acute investigations and can be managed by the patient and/or primary care team at home.[145]

Most exacerbations occur in and are treated in primary care. However, of these around 50% are thought not to be reported to the doctor either because patients deal with the exacerbation on

> *"For low oxygen flow rates, nasal prongs are convenient and simple to use and are usually more comfortable and less claustrophobic for patients"*

85

their own or because they do not classify their symptoms as an exacerbation.

During the winter months, symptoms are likely to deteriorate and exacerbations increase. This is probably linked to viral infection.[210] Symptoms, rather than lung function, deteriorate significantly before an exacerbation, and severe episodes often require hospitalization.

Exacerbations affect both lung function and symptoms, both of which affect a patient's general well being. However, it is the effect on lung function that is more detrimental to patients, with the evidence suggesting that each exacerbation hastens the rate of decline in lung

❝Most exacerbations occur in and are treated in primary care❞

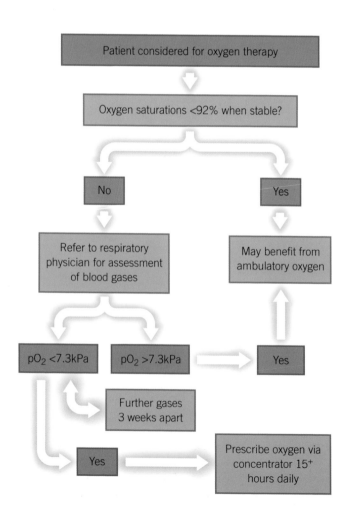

Fig. 49. Assessing the need for long-term oxygen therapy in patients with COPD.

function and that recovery from the exacerbation often does not lead to recovered lung function.[211]

Exacerbations also have an impact on health care resources. For example, during winter hospital admissions for COPD can augment the problem of bed shortages and lead to cancellations of surgical operations.

In an acute exacerbation, a patient may present with the following common symptoms:

- increased sputum purulence
- increased sputum volume
- wheeze

Primary	Secondary
• Tracheobronchial infection	• Pneumonia
• Air pollution	• Pulmonary embolism
	• Pneumothorax
	• Rib fractures/chest trauma
	• Inappropriate use of sedatives, narcotics, β-blockers
	• Right and/or left heart failure or arrhythmias

Fig. 50. Common causes of acute exacerbations of COPD.

- breathlessness
- chest tightness
- reduced exercise tolerance.

Why exacerbations occur is often unclear.[212] Common causes of acute exacerbations are listed in Figure 50. Previously, bacterial infections were thought to be the main cause, although at least one-third of cases are found to be the result of viral or non-infective sources.[213]

All patients with COPD suffer exacerbations to varying degrees, although they are more common in severe disease. There is considerable variation in the pattern of exacerbations. Many patients have three or more per year, while others have fewer.[212] In patients who experience frequent exacerbations, recovery time may be prolonged and the

“One-third of exacerbation cases are found to be due to viral or non-infective sources”

87

loss of lung function may not recover fully before the next exacerbation occurs. This contributes to more rapid progressive deterioration.

Treatment of exacerbations

By increasing bronchodilator use, either via an MDI with a spacer or, less frequently,[214] via a nebulizer many exacerbations can be treated at home. When there are signs of infection – as in the presence of excessive, purulent or green sputum – a short course of appropriate antibiotic can be prescribed.[145, 215] If the sputum remains white, antibiotics will not be required,[145] although they should be used if there is increased breathlessness. Increased breathlessness, or evidence of wheeze, is also an indication for a short course of oral steroids.[216]

"Patients with COPD who develop a cold may be prone to more severe exacerbations and should be considered for a short course of oral steroids"

Patients with COPD who develop a cold may be prone to more severe exacerbations and should be considered for a short course of oral steroid therapy at the onset of symptoms. Short courses of 7–10 days are advised as they are of most benefit during the first 72 hours of an exacerbation.[148,217].

Acute episodes that are followed-up or managed at home, can provide an opportunity to prevent further exacerbations and hospitalizations and help the patient plan for the future. Planned monitoring of the patient after discharge is essential for rehabilitation and encouraging self-management.

Home care is preferable if possible, but if a patient does not respond fully to treatment within 2 weeks of an exacerbation, referral for a chest radiograph or hospital appointment may be indicated.

Acute exacerbations that cannot be managed at home should be referred to secondary care.[145] Patients should be referred to hospital if any of the following are present:

"Many patients with COPD are repeatedly admitted to hospital and need to be empowered to cope"

- inability to cope at home (patient lives alone or carers cannot cope)
- severe breathlessness
- poor physical functioning
- cyanosis
- severe peripheral oedema
- impaired conscious level
- on long-term oxygen therapy
- rapid onset of exacerbation
- poor response to treatment.

Many patients with COPD are repeatedly admitted to hospital and need to be empowered to cope. Hospital treatment may be identical to that available at home. Home care and early discharge schemes aim to prevent and reduce levels of hospitalization.[218] While these schemes reduce the number of days patients spend in hospital, in general the level of home support required may be higher than that received in hospital, re-admission rates vary.[148] and the schemes are expensive.[219]

It is evident that patients need adequate support to be able to cope at home. Referral to secondary care may also occasionally be used to give the patient or the carer much needed respite, although the constant pressure on medical beds means this is often perceived as an inappropriate use of resources. Patients with COPD should be made more aware of the symptoms of an exacerbation and encouraged to report these early to clinicians.

Self-management plans

Early evidence suggests that personal COPD action plans may be effective. They are being evaluated.

Calculating the body mass index
BMI = weight in kg/(height in metres)^2

Fig. 51. How to calculate body mass index.

Non-pharmacological treatments
Pulmonary rehabilitation

Because COPD is progressive, managing patients with the condition often centres on controlling symptoms and acute exacerbations through optimal medication. However, drug therapy cannot address some of the loss of physical condition and social activity.

Although it does not alter the course of disease or survival, pulmonary rehabilitation – consisting of a structured programme of education, exercise, and physiotherapy – can improve exercise capacity, physical functioning, quality of life and enhance patients' sense of control over their condition.[224,225] Pulmonary rehabilitation can also reduce symptoms and use of health care[199,220–223] and may be generally useful for breaking the spiral of deconditioning and disability.

Pulmonary rehabilitation is unfortunately only available to a small proportion of patients in the UK who might benefit. Programmes have developed predominantly in secondary care, but there has been an increasing interest in primary-care-based rehabilitation.[148]

There are benefits and drawbacks of programmes in both settings, because patients may experience less group support in a primary care setting, but receive less individualized treatment in a secondary care programme. Patient preference should therefore be taken into account when choosing a programme. Moreover, making sure that the patient is motivated is essential to the success of pulmonary rehabilitation.[224,225]

The extent of rehabilitation that the primary care team can initiate depends on the severity of the COPD, body mass index (see Figure 51, page 89) and symptoms.

"Nutritional status is an important consideration in the overall care of patients with COPD"

Key aims for rehabilitation are as follows:

- strive for optimal symptomatic treatment
- offer or refer for smoking cessation programmes
- regularly check on inhalation technique
- provide advice on regular physical exercise
- provide access to dietician for patients with high or low BMI
- provide psychosocial and educational guidance via respiratory nurse or physician. A social worker can provide support for psychosocial, depression, social isolation or acceptance problems
- give advice on self-management skills – recognize any change in course of the disease, cough technique, medication compliance, nutrition or weight, adequate communication to the health care provider or insight into occupational factors.
- provide access to a specialized primary care physiotherapist for regular exercise training and breathing technique.

Diet and nutrition

Nutritional status is an important consideration in the overall care of patients with COPD. It has been estimated that approximately one-quarter of all COPD patients weigh less than 90% of their ideal.[226] Underweight patients are at risk of increased mortality.[148] The association between chronic respiratory disease and weight loss contributes toward a decline in lung function.[148]

"The association between chronic respiratory disease and weight loss contributes toward a decline in lung function"

The cause of weight loss in COPD is unclear, although the pattern of loss appears to be similar to that seen in malignant disease. COPD has systemic side-effects such as oxidative stress, abnormal levels of circulating cytokines, an increase in inflammatory cells and reduced skeletal mass, which are likely to contribute to weight loss.

Weight loss may be due to a combination of factors, such as an increased metabolic demand from the effort of breathing, or reduced dietary intake due to breathlessness and swallowing difficulties. Patients may lose interest in preparing food and lack enjoyment in their eating. These factors combine to make malnourishment very difficult to treat, so early detection and treatment are important.

Improved nutrition combined with a short course of anabolic steroids have been shown to improve lung function in patients with COPD.[227]

Monitoring weight is important and can be recorded simply as the patient's body mass index; the results can then be checked against a standard table (Figure 52) and documented in the patient's notes.

Dietary advice is just as important for patients who are overweight as additional weight can increase breathlessness. Assessing nutritional problems in COPD is complex because patients range from the underweight "pink puffer" to the overweight "blue bloater." Some patients may be clinically obese but nutritionally impaired.

The role of diet both in assisting the prevention of COPD and in preventing further deterioration is uncertain. Several epidemiological studies investigating the protective effect of antioxidants on lung function have found positive associations between low dietary intake of fruit and vegetables and decreased lung function in the general population.[228–230] Fruit and vegetable consumption appears to be inversely associated with development of COPD and it is postulated that diet might provide one explanation for differential development of COPD in smokers.[230]

66Of all the symptoms that patients with chronic respiratory disease experience, breathlessness is the most commonly reported and the most frightening and limiting for the patient 99

Treating dyspnoea

Of the many symptoms that patients with chronic respiratory disease experience, breathlessness is the most commonly reported and the most frightening and limiting for patients.

The degree and impact of breathlessness is not necessarily indicative of the severity of the underlying disease. Many patients with severe disease do not seem to experience breathlessness, while others who are at a milder stage of the disease process will be acutely aware of their breathing even on relatively minimal exertion, and they will experience breathlessness and the accompanying sensations.

Body mass index	Nutritional status
<16.0	Severe malnourishment
16.0–18.5	Moderate malnourishment
18.5–21.0	At risk of malnourishment
21.0–25.0	Ideal
25–30	Moderate obesity
>30.0	Severe obesity

Fig. 52. Nutritional status according to body mass index.

It is often the fear of becoming breathless that leads to inactivity, and this in turn leads to deconditioning, anxiety, loss of independence, helplessness and reduced self-esteem.

Useful home treatments for managing breathlessness include relaxation and physiotherapy. Occupational therapists can work with the patient on individual goal-setting and assess home ergonomics. The patient may need home aids such as perching stools, helping hands, bath and stair rails, chair lifts etc. An assessment by an occupational therapist in the patient's own home may conclude that the patient is able to manage his or her condition within the home setting. Home helps accessed through social services may assist with cleaning and shopping. Panic alarms or mobile phones may be useful and may help to counteract feelings of isolation for patients who live alone. Some patients may be living in unsuitable accommodation for managing their disease, and will need help and support in deciding on alternatives, such as moving to a bungalow, flat or sheltered housing. Any discussion about moving needs to be handled sensitively, as many people are very reluctant to move from their family home, however unsuitable it may be.

A useful measure for breathlessness is the Medical Research Council dyspnoea scale (Figure 53).

‎‎‎‎‎6‎6Patients with COPD may also have an underlying cardiac problem or there may be a malignancy 99

Other causes of dyspnoea

Patients with COPD may also have an underlying cardiac problem or there may be a malignancy. Evaluating the patient and making the correct diagnosis is important. For patients with cardiac problems, diuretics, angiotensin-converting enzyme (ACE) inhibitors and

Fig. 53. Medical Research Council dyspnoea scale.

Measuring breathlessness using the MRC dyspnoea scale
1   Not troubled by breathlessness unless on strenuous exercise
2   Short of breath when hurrying or walking up a slight hill
3   Walks slower than contemporaries on the level because of breathlessness or has to stop for breath when walking at own pace
4   Stops to take a breath after about 100m or a few minutes on the level
5   Too breathless to leave the house or breathless on dressing and undressing

digoxin may be useful. ACE inhibitors can cause cough in some patients. If there is an underlying malignancy, cytotoxic drugs and hormone therapy may help.

Non-specific dyspnoea

Where no specific cause for dyspnoea can be found, symptoms may be treated with drug therapies such as opioids, benzodiazepines, buspirone, antidepressants and cannabinoids.[256]

Psychological and social issues

Although there is considerable agreement on the treatment and management of COPD there are many patients whom, despite maximal medical treatment and pulmonary rehabilitation, still have problems. Current treatments, although valuable, are essentially palliative and there is insufficient evidence to conclude that any specific therapies alter the outcome of the disease.[148] Although survival may be an important goal, minimizing patient symptoms and improving the ability to function on a day-to-day basis may be more relevant to a patient's needs.[231] COPD is essentially a terminal disease although the process may be prolonged with a gradual deterioration.

Psychosocial support

Although symptom control is a substantial element in the care of chronic respiratory diseases, failure to address other aspects of the patient's life, such as behavioural responses, attitudes towards their disease and lifestyle, social and environmental factors, will lead to problems in coping with and adapting to the disease. Social support is an important part of human interaction and patients with a strong support network are more likely to have an enhanced health status and quality of life compared with individuals without support. The health care professional may be the main focus of support for some patients, yet there is little funding available for this.

The aims of psychosocial support are to:

- minimize the impact of the patient's disease on their lifestyle
- give support and reinforce the patient's own coping mechanisms
- allow for a degree of optimism and hope
- encourage the patient to use anxiety and panic management techniques
- encourage independence
- maximize the patient's potential.

Many patients with COPD feel they have failed. At a point in life when others may be looking forward to retirement, they find themselves with a chronic disease that does not improve but progressively

"Although survival may be an important goal, minimizing patient symptoms and improving the ability to function on a day-to-day basis may be more relevant to a patient's needs"

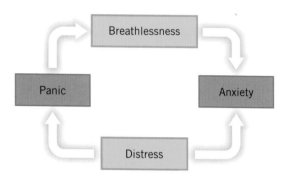

Fig. 54. The panic
cycle.

deteriorates. This impacts not only on the patient but also on their partners and families. Patients may suffer from guilt, feeling they have brought the disease upon themselves by actions such as smoking, and this unresolved guilt adds to their psychological overload. Negative emotions can increase the burden of physical problems.

In addition to a decline in their health patients also face other losses that are important to them, such as career, independence, role, responsibilities, relationship, hobbies and activities.

Anxiety and depression

Studies of psychological factors in patients with COPD indicate that anxiety, depression and selected psychiatric symptoms are common.[231–233] Data suggests a positive association between psychological distress and physical impairment, but there is a poor link between psychological and physiological functioning. Clearly psychological distress and poor self-image will impact on the patient's ability to undertake everyday activities. However, in some patients there are few, if any, psychological sequelae.[234] COPD is often also associated with poor body image, loneliness, reduced social support and negative self-concepts.[233,235]

The exact prevalence of anxiety and depression in COPD is unclear. Prevalence of anxiety appears to range from 2% to 34%,[231,236,237] and prevalence of depression appears to be around 42% in patients with moderate-to-severe COPD. Depression may be more prevalent in COPD than in other medical conditions. This is not surprising given the chronic progressive nature of the disease. Depression can be seen as a reasonable psychological response to the increasing limitations of the disease. Patients with COPD become increasingly housebound and can appear marginalized by the health care system.

Depressive symptoms are common in patients with severe disease, who have a 2.5 times greater risk.[243] It is important to be alert to symptoms of depression and treat appropriately.

> *Studies of psychological factors in patients with COPD indicate that anxiety, depression and selected psychiatric symptoms are common*

Anxiety and distress are linked to breathlessness. This leads to anxiety distress, which in turn leads to overbreathing and consequently breathlessness – the so-called panic cycle (Figure 54).

Strong emotions affect breathing and emotional stress can precipitate symptoms such as bronchospasm. It is often difficult to determine whether the emotions are the cause or effect of respiratory symptoms. Patients with COPD frequently use somatic complaints to cover their emotional concerns.[239]

The American College of Chest Physicians and the American Association of Cardiovascular and Pulmonary Rehabilitation[240] found little evidence that short-term psychosocial interventions work as single therapeutic modalities, but recognized that longer-term interventions may be beneficial. If a patient's psychosocial problems are minimized they become better at managing their disease and live longer.[241] The main aims of psychosocial support are shown in Figure 55.

66Strong emotions affect breathing and emotional stress can precipitate symptoms such as bronchospasm 99

Recognizing depression

The clinical features of depression are:
* crying and prolonged sadness
* loss of interest in and loss of enjoyment of life
* poor attention and concentration
* low self-esteem and ideas of unworthiness
* a bleak view of the future and the world in general
* poor sleep and appetite.

Useful treatments for depression and anxiety are:
* relaxation
* control of panic attacks
* breathing re-training

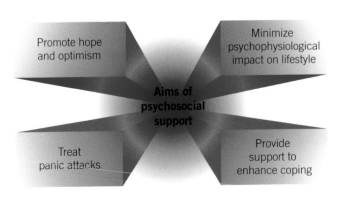

Fig. 55. Main aims of psychosocial support.

- teaching coping skills
- energy conservation
- psychological support
- increased activity, self-confidence and independence
- medication, such as antidepressants.

> *"Education is important for the COPD patient no matter what the stage of their disease"*

Education

Education is important at all stages of the disease. This may involve explaining the disease process, the use and purpose of medication for COPD and how to maintain health and independence. Advice should be given regularly about lifestyle changes and the importance of exercise.

Education will need to be adapted as the patient's condition deteriorates, and during times of crisis or exacerbation. It is important that long-term care is managed by a team who place the "expert patient" at the centre of management as this approach may help to maintain the patient's quality of life.[222]

Social factors

Around 44% of deaths from respiratory disease are associated with social class inequalities.[1] Social factors such as housing influence how the patient copes at home and their general and mental well-being.

Breathe Easy groups (see Appendix 4) offer social support and group interaction. For patients unable to attend meetings, newsletters and telephone helplines may be available. Local Age Concern groups (see Appendix 4) may also offer support, although availability varies geographically.

> *"44% of deaths from respiratory disease are associated with social class inequalities"*

Benefits

Simple advice on benefits and applications for "Blue badges" help the patient's independence and quality of life. The Benefits Agency has a helpline (see Appendix 4) for information on what benefits may be available.

Sexuality

An important issue associated with COPD that is infrequently discussed is sexuality and sexual relationships. Chronic lung disease impacts not only the sexual act itself, but also an individual's sexuality in the wider sense. Sexual problems are often mixed with problems of ageing, attitudes of the partner and breathlessness. By age 75 around 55% of men have experienced impotence problems.[242] The intimacy of a sexual relationship is important to everyone, but for patients with chronic lung disease sexual intimacy can be a powerful antidote to the depression and isolation associated with chronic illness.[225]

Although breathlessness is a major symptom of lung disease, studies show that this is not a major problem in sexual intercourse unless there is dyspnoea at rest.[243,244] Patients may have worries about inducing breathlessness but although breathing rate increases, the physical stress of sexual intercourse is comparable with climbing one or two flights of stairs and styles of love-making can vary considerably.[245]

Some patients may be concerned about sexual relationships so it is important to provide information or discuss the issue if it is a problem. The subject should be introduced with sensitivity, ensuring privacy and making referrals as necessary. General coping skills and sexual functioning are often linked in the chronically ill.

For the COPD patient, sexual activity is best performed:

- when rested
- slowly and surely
- after oxygen and bronchodilator medication
- thinking about positions that will reduce breathlessness
- focusing on the relationship itself rather than sexuality in isolation
- remembering to use all the senses and to experiment
- late morning/early afternoon
- not forgetting romance, kissing and cuddling
- with easily removable clothing
- avoiding alcohol, heavy meals and cigarette smoking
- remembering that orgasm is not the only goal.

Problems with intercourse can be indicative of problems that may need appropriate referral to other agencies, who are better equipped to deal with the issues.

The effect of medication on libido may be a useful starting point to discuss relationships with a patient. Medication may be the source of the problem or may be an aggravating factor. Common causes of impotence and reduced libido include antihypertensives, steroids, theophylline derivatives and anticholinergics.

Since many patients with chronic respiratory disease have systemic disease and take many medications, it is worth reviewing all prescription and over-the-counter drugs. While medication may be the solution to the physical problem, it will not provide the whole answer unless psychological and relationship difficulties have been addressed.[246]

> *"Of all diseases falling within the COPD disease category, emphysema is particularly progressive, leading to disabling dyspnoea and exercise limitation, with a substantial morbidity and reduced quality of life"*

Lung volume reduction surgery

Of all diseases falling within the COPD category, emphysema is particularly progressive, leading to disabling dyspnoea and exercise limitation, with a substantial morbidity and reduced quality of life. For a select group of patients with end-stage emphysema, lung volume reduction surgery (LVRS) may be beneficial.[247] LVRS appears to reduce dyspnoea, and improve lung function, exercise tolerance and health-related quality of life.[248] Larger trials are, however, required to assess the long-term treatment gains and perioperative mortality.[249]

LVRS is essentially a palliative, not a curative, procedure that takes the patient back to an earlier stage of the disease process.[248] LVRS may be unsuitable for certain patients with COPD, especially those with non-homogenous disease, severe lung obstruction and very severe parenchymal destruction.[247]

Palliative care

COPD is a terminal disease from the moment of diagnosis. Patients experience a slowly declining physical functioning that carries with it a concomitant effect on psychosocial function. Although palliative care is important throughout the development of the disease, there is inadequate provision. In the UK 75% of people die from non-malignant disease yet 95% of palliative care resources are used for the care of malignant disease.

Patients fear breathlessness and often feel they are going to die struggling for breath. The sensation of breathlessness is individual and derives from physiological, psychological, social and environmental factors that cause secondary physiological and behavioural responses.[250]

If the patient is anxious it is reasonable to use benzodiazepines. Dihydrocodeine and oral and parental opioids can be given on a trial basis.[251,252] There is no supporting evidence for nebulized opioids.[251,252]

Some practitioners may worry about addiction but in patients with an essentially terminal disease it is probably of little consequence.

Taking time to listen to a patient's concerns can help alleviate symptoms. Figure 56 summarizes the escalating care of the COPD patient.

> *"Patients fear breathlessness and often feel that they are going to die struggling for breath"*

Differential diagnoses and causes of dyspnoea

While the most common differential diagnosis for COPD is asthma, cardiac disease, tumour (tracheal, lung or laryngeal) bronchiectasis, foreign body, interstitial lung disease, pulmonary emboli, tuberculosis and aspiration are possibilities that should be investigated (Figure 57, page 100).

Future developments

With an increasing focus on COPD care and management, the next few years are likely to see significant advances. Prevention is the most important issue because once the pathological process is established, it cannot be reversed. An emphasis on early diagnosis and smoking cessation may help prevent development of moderate and severe disease. Improved structure of care, more regular reviews and pulmonary rehabilitation may help reduce the disability of COPD.

There has been interest in prescribing medication specifically tailored to COPD rather than relying on asthma therapy. Drugs that inhibit the enzyme phosphodiesterase type 4 can cause bronchodilation and inhibit neutrophilic inflammation. These drugs reduce

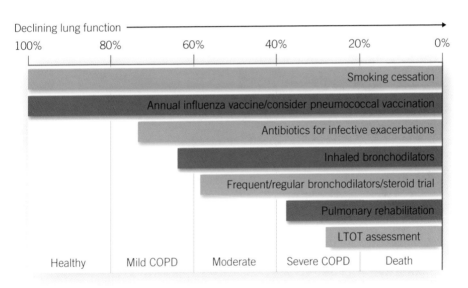

breathlessness, improve health and may reduce exacerbations, although so far they have caused transient gastrointestinal problems in a significant number of patients.[253]

Medications targeted at reducing mucus secretion or improving mucociliary clearance are also being developed.[148] In the future, mucolytic drugs may provide prophylaxis against exacerbations in patients with frequent or prolonged exacerbations as a result of hypersecretion of mucus.[254]

There are also several new anti-inflammatory drugs, specific mediator agonists, antiproteases, and pulmonary vasodilators, that might

Fig. 56. The escalator of care for COPD.

99

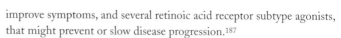

improve symptoms, and several retinoic acid receptor subtype agonists, that might prevent or slow disease progression.[187]

Increasingly research is focusing on cellular and molecular mechanisms that underlie the abnormal inflammatory response and may lead to new broad-spectrum anti-inflammatory drugs with a better safety profile than corticosteroids.[247]

Bronchoscopic volume reduction aims to decompress hyperinflated areas of lung, leading to symptomatic and functional improvement in patients with predominant emphysema, although peer review publications are awaited.[247]

Genetic factors are likely to be important for explaining why only a proportion of smokers develop COPD. Although smoking cessation is the only proven prophylactic measure, as drugs become more effective it will be possible to target therapeutic interventions towards predisposed patients before lung function is impaired.[188]

Fig. 57. Differential diagnosis of asthma and COPD.

Asthma	COPD
Affects all ages	Rarely seen under 40 years
No more common in smokers	More common in smokers
More common in those with atopy	Rarely runs in families without family history of asthma or familial alpha$_1$-antitrypsin deficiency
Chronic cough and sputum uncommon	Chronic cough and sputum common
Breathlessness intermittent and variable in severity	Breathlessness tends to be gradual and progressive
Primarily a disease of the more proximal and medium-sized bronchi	Primarily affects alveolar walls and smaller bronchi
Usually intermittent and paroxysmal	Usually a progressive, chronic disorder, producing daily symptoms
Airflow obstruction usually completely or partially reversible	Airflow obstruction fixed or only partially reversible
Good objective response to corticosteroid therapy	Poor objective response to corticosteroid therapy

Case study 1

Chronic bronchitis and emphysema

John, age 59, has a 45 pack-year smoking history. He had to take early retirement from the building trade because of increasing shortness of breath and presented at the surgery four times last winter with recurrent complaints of cough, purulent sputum and breathlessness.

On each visit to the practice, he was prescribed antibiotics by the GP and he claims that this improved his symptoms after 3 weeks.

Examination
John claims he was able to walk for 2 hours without undue breathlessness a year ago, but he is now increasingly breathless over short distances. He notices this is a problem when climbing stairs. His MRC dyspnoea score is 3 (see Figure 53, page 92).

John wakes at night but is unsure whether this is because of coughing or breathlessness. He has a "smoker's" cough, with phlegm that he claims is normally white. He has smoked 20 cigarettes a day since age 14.

" Because John has had frequent exacerbations, a 6-week trial of reversibility to steroids is suggested "

Investigations
Spirometry reveals an FEV_1 of 45% predicted, and a reduced FEV_1/FVC ratio. There is minimal reversibility on bronchodilation. Chest radiography is normal, although there is hyperinflation.

John's α_1-antitrypsin status should be considered for checking.

Diagnosis
The diagnosis is COPD.

Treatment plan
John should be prescribed bronchodilators, ideally long acting (anticholinergic or ß-agonist), with short-acting supplements and inhaled corticosteroids (in view of his history of repeated exacerbations). If an inadequate symptomatic response is achieved with one long-acting bronchodilator, then another class should be substituted or added.

The importance of smoking cessation should be stressed and psychological and therapeutic support should be offered. An action plan for future exacerbations should be agreed with John.

Ideally, pulmonary rehabilitation should be organized.

101

Case study 2
Asthma or depression?

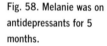

" *Melanie has talked to her partner about needing increased support* **"**

Melanie comes to the surgery for an asthma review because of continual troublesome symptoms. She is age 30 and claims to have had a cough for 3 months. She is increasingly short of breath. There appears to be no pattern to her symptoms, although she says that changes in temperature trigger the symptoms. She has a 12-year smoking history of around 25 cigarettes a day giving her a 15 pack-year history. She is stressed and tearful. Previously she was on antidepressants for five months but she stopped taking them four months ago. Her current medication is salbutamol 100 mcg prn and beclomethasone 100 mcg, 2 puffs twice daily.

Family history

Fig. 58. Melanie was on antidepressants for 5 months.

Both Melanie's maternal grandparents had asthma, but there is no parental or sibling history. Melanie does not have hayfever or eczema or any allegies. She has had an ear infection twice.

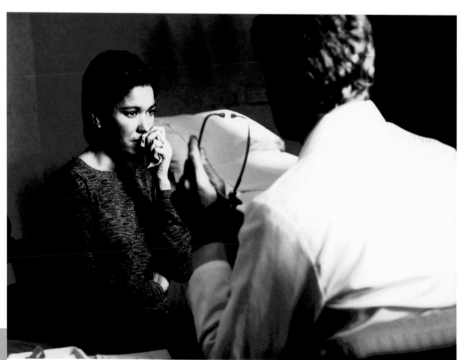

Social history

Melanie is married with no children. Her inhaler technique is good. Her peak expiratory flow rate of 280–450 l/min appears to have diurnal variation; her best peak expiratory flow rate is 450 l/min. This was discussed at the consultation, as was Aerochamber use for inhaled corticosteroids. The use of antidepressants was also discussed.

At 1-monthly review

Melanie says she feels better. She started taking paroxetine 20 mg od, and still has some symptoms, although salbutamol use is minimal. Melanie has talked to her partner about needing increased support. Her PEF is still 350–450 l/min. She is asked to try a LABA in addition to her inhaled steroid.

Further 1-monthly review

Melanie feels well and has stopped paroxetine and all her inhalers. She stopped smoking 1 month ago by going "cold turkey".She recently bought a new car. No peak expiratory flow charts were available, but spirometry revealed an FEV_1 of 97%, an FVC of 99%and an FEV_1/FVC ratio of 97%.

Treatment plan

Although Melanie feels well and is proud that she has gone "cold turkey", because her previous PEF showed diurnal variation and symptoms she will need ongoing support. She should be reviewed to ensure she remains symptom-free and advised to consult if she experiences symptoms in the future.

« Although Melanie feels well and is proud that she has gone cold turkey, she will need ongoing support »

Case study 3
Asthma in a child

Andrew is age 5 and was diagnosed as having asthma 2 years ago when he had a persistent nocturnal cough. The trigger factors for his asthma are cats and house dust mites. The cat has been re-housed and Andrew's mother has put mattress protectors on her son's bed. His grandfather has asthma. Andrew was small for dates but looked well.

" Andrew's inhaler devices should be rationalized "

Current medication
Andrew is asymptomatic. His inhaler technique is good but fast. His current medication is:

* Sodium cromoglicate 5 mg 2 puffs twice daily with a Fisonair device
* Beclomethasone 50 mcg 2 puffs twice daily using an Aerochamber
* Salbutamol 1–2 puffs three times daily via a Volumatic.

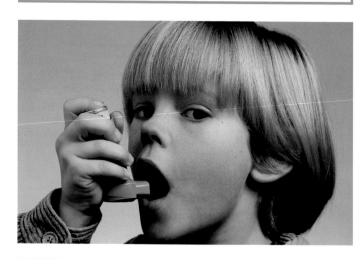

Fig. 59. Andrew's inhaler technique is good but fast

Treatment plan
Andrew should reduce his cromoglicate therapy to 1 puff twice daily for 2 weeks. He should stop altogether if his symptoms do not reappear. He should then be given salbutamol on an "as required" basis. Andrew's inhaler devices should be rationalized.

His GP should consider prescribing a leukotriene receptor antagonist or a LABA in addition to his inhaled steroid if symptoms recur.

Short-acting β₂-agonists for asthma

Drug	Format	Trade names	Preparation	Strengths	Doses used in asthma	Comments	Side-effects
Salbutamol	Inhaled	Generic	MDI	100mcg	100-200mcg 3-4 times/d; child 100mcg 3-4 times/d	Inhaled salbutamol is the drug of choice for acute bronchospasm, and should be taken as needed	Tremor, tachycardia (especially with nebulized preparations)
			DPI	200mcg, 400mcg	200-400mcg 3-4 times/d; child 200mcg 3-4 times/d		
			Nebulizer solution	1mg/ml; 2mg/ml	2.5-5mg 3-4 times/d	The inhaled route is more effective than the oral route	
		Aerolin Autohaler	BAMDI	100mcg	100-200mcg 3-4 times/d; child 100mcg 3-4 times/d	Inhaled salbutamol should ideally be delivered via an oxygen-driven nebulizer in the emergency setting	
		Airomir Inhaler	MDI	100mcg	100-200mcg 3-4 times/d; child 100mcg 3-4 times/d		
		Airomir Autohaler	BAMDI	100mcg	100-200mcg 3-4 times/d; child 100mcg 3-4 times/d		
		Asmasal Clickhaler	DPI	95mcg	95-190mcg 3-4 times/d; child 95mcg 3-4 times/d	MDIs and spacers have been shown to be as effective as nebulisers in many studies	
		Salamol Easi-Breathe Inhaler	BAMDI	100mcg	100-200mcg 3-4 times/d; child 100mcg 3-4 times/d		
		Ventodisks	DPI	200mcg, 400mcg	200-400mcg 3-4 times/d; child 200mcg 3-4 times/d		
		Ventolin Evohaler	MDI	100mcg	100-200mcg 3-4 times/d; child 100mcg 3-4 times/d		
		Ventolin Accuhaler	DPI	200mcg	200mcg 3-4 times/d		
		Ventolin Nebules	Nebuliser solution	1mg/ml, 2mg/ml	2.5-5mg 3-4 times/d		
		Ventolin Respirator Solution	Nebuliser solution	5mg/ml	2.5-5mg 3-4 times/d	Dilute with sterile sodium chloride 0.9%	

Short-acting β₂-agonists for asthma

Drug	Format	Trade names	Preparation	Strengths	Doses used in asthma	Comments	Side-effects
Salbutamol	Oral	Generic	Tablet	2mg, 4mg	2-4mg 3-4 times/d; child 2-6 years 1-2mg 3-4 times/d, 6-12 years 2mg 3-4 times/d	Oral salbutamol is no longer recommended for the treatment of asthma	Tremor, tachycardia (especially with nebulized preparations)
			Oral solution	2mg/5ml	2-4mg 3-4 times/d; child 2-6 years 1-2mg 3-4 times/d, 6-12 years 2mg 3-4 times/d		
		Ventmax SR	M/R capsule	4mg, 8mg	8mg 2 times/d; child 3-12 years 4mg 2 times/d		
		Ventolin	Syrup	2mg/5ml	2-4mg 3-4 times/d; child 2-6 years 1-2mg 3-4 times/d, 6-12 years 2mg 3-4 times/d		
		Volmax	Tablet	4mg, 8mg	8mg 2 times/d; child 3-12 years 4mg 2 times/d		
Terbutaline	Inhaled	Generic	Nebulizer solution	2.5mg/ml	5-10mg 2-4 times/d; child < 3 years 2mg 2-4 times/d, 3-6 years 3mg 2-4 times/d, 6-8 years 4mg 2-4 times/d, > 8years 5mg 2-4 times/d		Tremor, tachycardia (especially with nebulized preparations)
		Bricanyl Inhaler	MDI	250mcg	250-500mcg 3-4 times/d		
		Bricanyl Turbohaler	DPI	500mcg	250-500mcg 3-4 times/d		
		Bricanyl Respules	Nebulizer solution	2.5mg/ml	5-10mg 2-4 times/d; child < 3 years 2mg 2-4 times/d, 3-6 years 3mg 2-4 times/d, 6-8 years 4mg 2-4 times/d, > 8years 5mg 2-4 times/d		
		Bricanyl Respirator Solution	Nebulizer solution	10mg/ml	5-10mg 2-4 times/d; child < 3 years 2mg 2-4 times/d, 3-6 years 3mg 2-4 times/d, 6-8 years 4mg 2-4 times/d, > 8years 5mg 2-4 times/d	Dilute with sterile sodium chloride 0.9%	

Short-acting β₂-agonists for asthma

Drug	Format	Trade names	Preparation	Strengths	Doses used in asthma	Comments	Side-effects
Terbutaline	Oral	Bricanyl	Tablet	5mg	2.5-5mg 3 times/d; child 7-15 years 2.5mg 2-3 times/d	Not recommended	Tremor, tachycardia, hyperkalaemia
			Syrup	1.5mg/5ml	2.5-5mg 3 times/d; child <7years 75mcg/kg 3 times/d, 7-15 years 2.5mg 2-3 times/d		
		Bricanyl SA	M/R tablet	7.5mg	7.5mg 2 times/d		
		Monovent	Syrup	1.5mg/5ml	2.5-5mg 3 times/d; child <7years 75mcg/kg 3 times/d, 7-15 years 2.5mg 2-3 times/d		
Fenoterol + ipratropium	Inhaled	Duovent Nebulizer Solution	Nebulizer solution	1.25mg + 500mcg/4ml	1 vial up to 4 times daily; not recommended for children < 14 years	Combination products are only recommended if compliance is a problem	Tremor, tachycardia (especially with nebulizedpreparations), dry mouth, urinary retention, constipation, blurred vision, risk of glaucoma with nebulized formulations

Long-acting β₂-agonists for asthma

Drug	Format	Trade names	Preparation	Strengths	Doses used in asthma	Comments	Side-effects
Bambuterol	Oral	Bambec	Tablet	10mg, 20mg	10-20mg nocte; not recommended for children	Not recommended	Tremor, tachycardia, hyperkalaemia
Formoterol	Inhaled	Foradil	DPI	12mcg	12-24mcg 2 times/d; not recommended for children < 5 years	Not for relief of acute asthma attacks	Tremor, tachycardia, hyperkalaemia
		Oxis	DPI	6mcg, 12mcg	6-24mcg 1-2 times/d (max 36mg 2 times/d) child > 6 years 12mcg 1-2 times/d		
Salmeterol	Inhaled	Serevent Inhaler	MDI	25mcg	50-100mcg 2 times/d; child > 4 years 50mcg 2 times/d	Not for relief of acute asthma attacks	Tremor, tachycardia, paradoxical bronchospasm, hyperkalaemia
		Serevent Accuhaler	DPI	50mcg	50-100mcg 2 times/d; child > 4 years 50mcg 2 times/d		
		Serevent Diskhaler	DPI	50mcg	50-100mcg 2 times/d; child > 4 years 50mcg 2 times/d		

107

Anticholinergic bronchodilators for asthma

Drug	Format	Trade names	Preparation	Strengths	Doses used in asthma	Comments	Side-effects
Ipratropium	Inhaled	Generic	Nebulizer solution	250mcg/ml	100-500mcg up to 4 times/d; child 3-14 years 100-500mcg up to 3 times/d	Anticholinergic bronchodilators are an alternative reliever medication for patients who cannot tolerate β_2 agonists. They may provide additional benefits but have a slower onset of action	Dry mouth, urinary retention, constipation, blurred vision, risk of glaucoma with nebulized formulations (especially when given with salbutamol)
		Atrovent Inhaler	MDI	20mcg, 40mcg	20-80mcg 3-4 times/d; child < 6 years 20mcg 3 times/d, 6-12 years 20-40mcg 3 times/d		
		Atrovent Aerocaps	DPI	40mcg	40-80mcg 3 times/d; not recommended for children < 12 years		
		Atrovent Autohaler	BAMDI	20mcg	20-80mcg 3-4 times/d; child < 6 years 20mcg 3 times/d, 6-12 years 20-40mcg 3 times/d	The evidence for their effect in young children is marginal and there is insufficient evidence to support the uncritical use of anticholinergics in infants	
		Atrovent Nebulizer Solution	Nebulizer solution	250mcg/ml	100-500mcg up to 4 times/d; child 3-14 years 100-500mcg up to 3 times/d		
		Respontin	Nebulizer solution	250mcg/ml	100-500mcg up to 4 times/d; child 3-14 years 100-500mcg up to 3 times/d	Used to manage chronic asthma in patients who require high doses of corticosteroids	

Methylxanthines for asthma

Drug	Format	Trade names	Preparation	Strengths	Doses used in asthma	Comments	Side-effects
Theophylline	Oral	Nuelin	Tablet	125mg	125-250mg 3-4 times/d; child 7-12 years 62.5-125mg 3-4 times/d	Formulations are not interchangeable; take after food and swallow whole	**Plasma concentrations must be monitored;** multiple interactions with other drugs; nausea, tachycardia, hypokalaemia
			Liquid	60mg/5ml	120-240mg 3-4 times/d; child 2-6 years 60-90mg 3-4 times/d, 7-12 years 90-120mg 3-4 times/d	Methylxanthines are an option for add-on treatment in patients with moderate-to-severe persistent asthma. Not recommended as first choice because of the difficulty in titrating individual dosage and the high occurrence of potentially serious side-effects	Nausea and vomiting are most common. Serious effects occurring at higher serum concentrations include seizures, tachycardia, and arrhythmias
		Nuelin SA	M/R tablet	175mg, 250mg	175-500mg 2 times/d; child > 6 years 125-250mg 2 times/d		
		Slo-Phyllin	M/R capsule	60mg, 125mg, 250mg	250-500mg 2 times/d; child 2-6 years 60-120mg 2 times/d, 7-12 years 125-250mg		

Methylxanthines for asthma

Drug	Format	Trade names	Preparation	Strengths	Doses used in asthma	Comments	Side-effects
Theophylline	Oral	Uniphyllin Continus	M/R tablet	200mg, 300mg, 400mg	200-400mg 2 times/d; child >7 years 9mg/kg 2 times/d (max 10-16mg/kg 2 times/d)		
Aminophylline	Oral	Generic	Tablet	100mg	100-300mg 3-4 times/d	Formulations are not interchangeable; take after food and swallow whole	**Plasma concentrations must be monitored;** multiple interactions with other drugs; nausea, tachycardia, hypokalaemia
		Phyllocontin Continus	M/R tablet	100mg, 225mg, 350mg	225-450mg 2 times/d; smokers 350-700mg 2 times/d; child > 3 years 6-12 mg/kg 2 times/d (max 13-20mg/kg 2 times/d)		

Corticosteroids for asthma

Drug	Format	Trade names	Preparation	Strengths	Doses used in asthma	Comments	Side-effects
Beclometasone	Inhaled	Generic	MDI	50mcg, 100mcg, 200mcg, 250mcg	200mcg 2 times/d or 100mcg 3-4 times/d (initially 600-800mcg/d in patients with severe asthma; max 500mcg 4 times/d); child 50-100mcg 2-4 times/d	Used to manage chronic asthma not controlled by short-acting B₂ stimulants	Oropharyngeal candidiasis, paradoxical bronchospasm, easy bruising, osteoporosis, cataracts (side-effects are dose- and duration dependent)
			DPI	100mcg, 200mcg, 400mcg	400mcg 2 times/d or 200mcg 3-4 times/d (max 800mcg 2 times/d); child 100mcg 2-4 times/d or 200mcg 2 times/d		Side-effects are very rare at low doses (up to 800mcg (400mcg in children) beclomethasone or equivalent daily). At higher doses may cause a range of side-effects including skin thinning and bruises, and rarely adrenal suppression
		AeroBec Autohaler	BAMDI	50mcg, 100mcg, 250mg	200mcg 2 times/d or 100mcg 3-4 times/d (initially 600-800mcg/d in patients with severe asthma; max 500mcg 4 times/d); child 50-100mcg 2-4 times/d		
		Asmabec Clickhaler	DPI	50mcg, 100mcg, 250mcg	200-400mcg in 2-4 divided doses (initially 0.8-1.6mg in 2-4 divided doses in patients with severe asthma; max 500mcg 4 times/d); child 50-100mcg 2-4 times/d		
		Beclazone Easi-Breathe Inhaler	BAMDI	50mcg, 100mcg, 250mcg	200mcg 2 times/d or 100mcg 3-4 times/d (initially 600-800mcg/d in patients with severe asthma; max 500mcg 4 times/d); child 50-100mcg 2-4 times/d		

Corticosteroids for asthma

Drug	Format	Trade names	Preparation	Strengths	Doses used in asthma	Comments	Side-effects
Beclometasone	Inhaled	Becodisks	DPI	100mcg, 200mcg, 400mcg	400mcg 2 times/d or 200mcg 3-4 times/d (max 800mcg 2 times/d); child 100mcg 2-4 times/d or 200mcg 2 times/d		Local side-effects include hoarseness and oropharyngeal candidiasis (using spacer devices with MDIs and washing the mouth after using DPIs decrease this side-effect). Minor growth delay or suppression (average 1cm) in children has also been observed at medium and high doses, but attainment of predicted adult height does not appear to be affected. Use for all inhaled steroids
		Becotide and Becloforte Inhalers	MDI	50mcg, 100mcg, 200mcg, 250mcg	200mcg 2 times/d or 100mcg 3-4 times/d (initially 600-800mcg/d in patients with severe asthma; max 500mcg 4 times/d); child 50-100mcg 2-4 times/d		
		Qvar Inhaler	MDI	50mcg, 100mcg	50-200mcg 2 times/d (max 400mcg 2 times/d); not recommended for children	Lower doses of beclomethasone are given because of the propellant used in these formulations	
		Qvar Autohaler	BAMDI	50mcg,	50-200mcg 2 times/d (max 400mcg 2 times/d); not recommended for children		
Budesonide	Inhaled	Generic	DPI	200mcg, 400mcg	200-400mcg every evening (max 800mcg 2 times/d in severe asthma); child < 12 years 100-200mcg 2 times/d (max 400mcg 2 times/d in severe asthma) or 200-400mcg every evening	Used to manage chronic asthma not controlled by short-acting B_2 stimulants	Oropharyngeal candidiasis, paradoxical bronchospasm, easy bruising, osteoporosis, cataracts (side-effects are dose- and duration dependent)
		Pulmicort Inhaler	MDI	50mcg, 200mcg	200-400mcg 2 times/d (max 1.6mg/d in severe asthma); child 50-400mcg 2 times/d (max 800mcg/d in severe asthma)		
		Pulmicort Turbohaler	DPI	100mcg, 200mcg, 400mcg	200-400mcg every evening (max 800mcg 2 times/d in severe asthma); child < 12 years 100-200mcg 2 times/d (max 400mcg 2 times/d in severe asthma) or 200-400mcg every evening		
		Pulmicort Respules	Nebulizer suspension	250mcg/ml	0.5-1mg 2 times/d (1-2mg 2 times/d in severe asthma); child 3 months to 12 years 250-500mcg 2 times/d (0.5-1mg 2 times/d in severe asthma)		

Corticosteroids for asthma

Drug	Format	Trade names	Preparation	Strengths	Doses used in asthma	Comments	Side-effects
Fluticasone	Inhaled	Flixotide Evohaler	MDI	25mcg, 50mcg, 125mcg, 250mcg	100-250mcg 2 times/d (max 1mg 2 times/d); child 4-16 years 50-100mcg 2 times/d (max 200mcg 2 times/d)	Used to manage chronic asthma not controlled by short-acting β₂ stimulants	Oropharyngeal candidiasis, paradoxical bronchospasm, easy bruising, osteoporosis, cataracts (side-effects are dose- and duration dependent)
		Flixotide Accuhaler	DPI	50mcg, 100mcg, 250mcg, 500mcg	100-250mcg 2 times/d (max 1mg 2 times/d); child 4-16 years 50-100mcg 2 times/d (max 200mcg 2 times/d)		
		Flixotide Diskhaler	DPI	50mcg, 100mcg, 250mcg, 500mcg	100-250mcg 2 times/d (max 1mg 2 times/d); child 4-16 years 50-100mcg 2 times/d (max 200mcg 2 times/d)		
		Flixotide Nebules	Nebulizer suspension	250mcg/ml	0.5-2mg 2 times/d;	Not recommended for children	
Mometasone	Inhaled	Asmanex Twisthaler	DPI	200mcg, 400mcg	200-400mcg 1 time/d in the evening, or in 2 divided doses. Dose increased to 400mcg twice daily if necessary	Not recommended for children	Oral candidiasis, dysphonia, pharyngitis, headache, systemic corticosteroid effects, hypersensitivity reactions
Prednisolone	Oral	Generic	Tablet	1mg, 5mg	30-60mg/d taken in the morning after breakfast for a few days to control acute asthma attacks; reduce dose gradually if asthma control is poor	Use high-dose inhaled corticosteroids when possible as they have fewer side-effects	Gastrointestinal (dyspepsia, ulceration), musculoskeletal (osteoporosis), endocrine (adrenal suppression), cushingoid effects likely with prolonged dosing >7.5mg/d, weight gain), neuropsychiatric (euphoria, depression), ophthalmic (glaucoma, cataracts)
			E/C tablet	2.5mg, 5mg			
			Soluble tablet	5mg			
		Deltacortril	E/C tablet	2.5mg, 5mg			
		Precortisyl Forte	Tablet	25mg			

Combined corticosteroids and long-acting β-agonists for asthma

Drug	Format	Trade names	Preparation	Strengths	Doses used in asthma	Comments	Side-effects
Budesonide + formoterol	Inhaled	Symbicort Turbohaler	DPI	80mcg + 4.5mcg; 160mcg + 4.5mcg	1-2 puffs 1-2 times/d; not recommended for children and adolescents < 17 years	Used to manage chronic asthma not controlled by short-acting β₂ stimulants	Oropharyngeal candidiasis, paradoxical bronchospasm, easy bruising, osteoporosis, cataracts (side-effects are dose- and duration dependent), tremor, tachycardia, hypokalaemia
Fluticasone + salmeterol	Inhaled	Seretide Evohaler	MDI	50mcg + 25mcg; 125mcg + 25mcg; 250mcg + 25mcg	100mcg + 50mcg to 500mcg + 50mcg 2 times/d reducing dose to once daily if control of asthma is maintained; not recommended for children < 12 years old	Used to manage chronic asthma not controlled by short-acting β₂ stimulants; combination products are only recommended if compliance is a problem	Oropharyngeal candidiasis, paradoxical bronchospasm, easy bruising, osteoporosis, cataracts (side-effects are dose- and duration dependent), tremor, tachycardia, hyperkalaemia
		Seretide Accuhaler	DPI	100mcg + 50mcg; 250mcg + 50mcg; 500mcg + 50mcg	100mcg + 50mcg to 500mcg + 50mcg 2 times/d reducing dose to once daily if control of asthma is maintained; not recommended for children < 12 years old		

Cromoglicate and related therapy for asthma

Drug	Format	Trade names	Preparation	Strengths	Doses used in asthma	Comments	Side-effects
Sodium cromoglicate	Inhaled	Generic	MDI	5mg	10mg 4 times/d (max 10mg 6-8 times/d)	There is minimal evidence of effectiveness either as a sole controller therapy or as an add-on to inhaled steroids. Use should be limited to specialist practice	Coughing, transient bronchospasm and throat irritation
			Nebulizer solution	10mg/ml	20mg 4 times/d (max 20mg 6 times/d)		
		Cromogen Easi-Breathe Inhaler	MDI	5mg	10mg 4 times/d (max 10mg 6-8 times/d)		
		Intal Inhaler	MDI	5mg	10mg 4 times/d (max 10mg 6-8 times/d)		
		Intal Spincaps	DPI	20mg	20mg 4 times/d (max 8 times/d)		
		Intal Nebulizer Solution	Nebulizer solution	10mg/ml	20mg 4 times/d (max 20mg 6 times/d)		

Cromoglicate and related therapy for asthma

Drug	Format	Trade names	Preparation	Strengths	Doses used in asthma	Comments	Side-effects
Sodium cromoglicate + salbutamol	Inhaled	Aerocrom Inhaler	MDI	1mg + 100mcg	2 puffs 4 times/d; not recommended for children	Not recommended	Coughing, transient bronchospasm and throat irritation, tremor, tachycardia, hyperkalaemia
Nedocromil sodium	Inhaled	Tilade Inhaler	MDI	2mg	4mg 4 times/d; not recommended for children > 6 years	There is minimal evidence of effectiveness either as a sole controller therapy or as add-on to inhaled steroids. Use should be limited to specialist practice	Coughing, transient bronchospasm and throat irritation

Ketotifen for asthma

Drug	Format	Trade names	Preparation	Strengths	Doses used in asthma	Comments	Side-effects
Ketotifen	Oral	Zaditen	Capsule	1mg	1-2mg 2 times/d; child > 2 years 1mg 2 times/d	Not recommended	Drowsiness, dry mouth, dizziness, CNS stimulation, weight gain
			Tablet	1mg	1-2mg 2 times/d; child > 2 years 1mg 2 times/d		
			Elixir	1mg/5ml	1-2mg 2 times/d; child > 2 years 1mg 2 times/d		

Leukotriene receptor antagonists for asthma

Drug	Format	Trade names	Preparation	Strengths	Doses used in asthma	Comments	Side-effects
Montelukast	Oral	Singulair	Chewable tablet	4mg, 5mg	10mg nocte; child 2-5 years 4mg nocte, 6-14 years 5mg nocte	Licensed as monotherapy for asthma associated with exercise, and as add-on therapy for symptomatic patients on inhaled corticosteroids	No specific adverse effects to date at recommended doses
			Tablet	10mg	10mg nocte; child 2-5 years 4mg nocte, 6-14 years 5mg nocte		
Zafirlukast	Oral	Accolate	Tablet	20mg	20mg 2 times daily; not recommended for children < 12 years	Not effective in relieving acute asthma attacks but used in prophylaxis of asthma	Elevation of liver enzymes

Short-acting β₂-agonists for COPD

Drug	Format	Trade names	Preparation	Strengths	Doses used in COPD	Comments	Side-effects
Salbutamol	Inhaled	Generic	MDI	100mcg	200mcg 3-4 times/d	Inhaled salbutamol should be used as needed or regularly to relieve breathlessness and improve exercise capacity	Tremor, tachycardia (especially with nebulized preparations)
			Nebulizer solution	1mg/ml, 2mg/ml	2.5-5mg 3-4 times/d		
		Aerolin Autohaler	BAMDI	100mcg	200mcg 3-4 times/d		
		Airomir	MDI	100mcg	200mcg 3-4 times/d		
			BAMDI	100mcg	200mcg 3-4 times/d		
		Asmasal Clickhaler	DPI	95 mcg	180mcg 3-4 times/d		
		Ventodisks	DPI	200mcg	200mcg 3-4 times/d		
		Ventolin	MDI	100mcg	200mcg 3-4 times/d	Most rapid onset of action of any class of bronchodilators; duration of action is 4-6 hours	
			Accuhaler	200mcg	200mcg 3-4 times/d		
			Salamol Easi-Breathe inhaler	100mcg	200mcg 3-4 times/d		
			Nebules	2.5mg, 5 mg	2.5-5mg 3-4 times/d	β-agonists act directly on bronchial smooth muscle to cause bronchodilatation. The dose response in patients with COPD is almost flat so there is little benefit in giving more than 1mg salbutamol or equivalent	
	Oral	Generic	Tablet	2mg, 4mg	2-4mg 3-4 times/d	Not recommended	Tremor, tachycardia, hypokalaemia
		Ventmax SR	Capsule	4mg	4-8mg 2 times/d		
		Ventolin	Syrup	2mg/5ml	2-4mg 3-4 times/d		
		Volmax	Tablet	4mg, 8mg	4-8mg 2 times/d		

Short-acting ß₂-agonists for COPD

Drug	Format	Trade names	Preparation	Strengths	Doses used in COPD	Comments	Side-effects
Terbutaline	Inhaled	Generic	Nebulizer solution	2.5mg/ml	5-10mg 3-4 times/d		Tremor, tachycardia (especially with nebulized preparations)
		Bricanyl	MDI	250mcg	250-500mcg 3-4times/d		
			Turbohlaler	500mcg	500mcg 3-4 times/d		
			Respules	2.5mg	5-10mg 3-4 times/d		
			Nebulizer solution	10mg/ml	5-10mg 3-4 times/d	Dilute with saline	
	Oral	Bricanyl	Tablets	5mg	2.5-5mg 3 times/d	Not recommended	Tremor, tachycardia, hypokalaemia
			Syrup	1.5mg/5ml	2.5-5mg 3 times/d		
		Bricanyl SA	Tablet	7.5mg	7.5mg 2 times/d		
		Monovent	Syrup	1.5mg/5ml	2.5-5mg 3 times/d		

Long-acting ß₂-agonists for COPD

Drug	Format	Trade names	Preparation	Strengths	Doses used in COPD	Comments	Side-effects
Bambuterol	Oral	Bambec	Tablet	10mg	10-20mg at night	Not recommended	Tremor, tachycardia, hypokalaemia
Formoterol	Inhaled	Foradil	Dry powder capsules	12mcg	12-24mcg 2 times/d	Rapid onset of action	Tremor, tachycardia, hypokalaemia
		Oxis	Turbohaler	6mcg, 12 mcg	6-24mcg 1-2 times/d		
Salmeterol	Inhaled	Serevent	MDI	25mcg	50-100mcg 2 times/d	Slow (>20 min) onset of action	Tremor, tachycardia, hypokalaemia, paradoxiacal bronchospasms
			Accuhaler	50mcg	50-100mcg 2 times/d	The bronchodilator effects of long-acting ß-agonists are similar to the short-acting agents, but their duration of action is about 12 hours. Studies show improved quality of life and symptoms, and some show a reduction in exacerbations	
			Diskhaler	50mcg	50-100mcg 2 times/d		

Anticholinergic bronchodilators for COPD

Drug	Format	Trade names	Preparation	Strengths	Doses used in COPD	Comments	Side-effects
Ipratropium	Inhaled	Generic	Nebulizer solution	250mcg/ml	250-500mcg 3-4 times/d	Anticholinergic drugs cause bronchodilatation by blocking muscarinic receptors and thereby the resting bronchoconstrictor tone induced by cholinergic nerves. Cholinergic nerves also mediate effects on mucus secretion	Dry mouth, urinary retention (rare), blurring of vision
		Atrovent	MDI	20mcg, 40mcg	40-80mcg 3-4 times/d		
			BAMDI	20mcg	40-80mcg 3-4 times/d		
			DPI	40mcg	40-80mcg 3-4 times/d		
			Nebulizer Solution	250mcg/ml	250-500mcg 3-4 times/d		
		Respontin	Nebulizer Solution	250mcg/ml	250-500mcg 3-4 times/d	Slightly longer acting than ipratropium (be aware this may be withdrawn)	Dry mouth, urinary retention (rare)

Once daily long-acting anticholinergic bronchodilators for COPD

Drug	Format	Trade names	Preparation	Strengths	Doses used in COPD	Comments	Side-effects
Tiotropium	Inhaled	Spiriva	DPI	18mcg	18mcg 1 time/d	Tiotropium is currently the only long-acting anticholinergic bronchodilator available. Its duration of action is such that it can be given once daily. It provides sustained benefits over one year in terms of lung function improvement, exercise tolerance, quality-of-life improvement and reduced exacerbations. It appears to be more effective than regular short-acting anticholinergic therapy	Dry mouth, urinary retention (rare), blurring of vision

Methylxanthines for COPD

Drug	Format	Trade names	Preparation	Strengths	Doses used in COPD	Comments	Side-effects
Theophylline	Oral	Nuelin	Tablet	125mg	125mg 3-4 times/d	Preparations are not interchangeable	**Plasma levels must be monitored** Multiple interactions with other drugs, nausea, tachycardia, hypokalaemia
			Syrup	60mg/5ml	120-240mg 3-4 times/d	The mechanism of action of these drugs remains uncertain, but it is thought they relax airway smooth muscle and have lesser beneficial effects by increasing diaphragmatic strength, improving mucociliary clearance and improving cardiac output. Because of potential toxicity and significant interactions with other drugs theophylline is no longer considered first-line treatment	
		Neulin SA	M/R tablet	175mg, 250mg	175-500mg 2 times/d		
		Slo-Phyllin	M/R capsule	60mg, 125mg, 250mg	250-500mg 2 times/d		
		Uniphyllin Continus	M/R tablet	200mg, 300mg, 400mg	200-400mg 2 times/d		
Aminophylline	Oral	Generic	Tablet	100mg	100-300mg 3-4 times/d	Preparations are not interchangeable	**Plasma levels must be monitored** Multiple interactions with other drugs, nausea, tachycardia, hypokalaemia
		Phyllocontin Continus	M/R tablet	225mg, 350mg	225-750mg 2 times/d		

Corticosteroids for COPD

Drug	Format	Trade names	Preparation	Strengths	Doses used in COPD	Comments	Side-effects
Beclometasone	Inhaled	Generic	MDI	50mcg, 100mcg, 200mcg, 250mcg	100-800mcg 2 times/d	While there is no clear mechanism for effectiveness of these drugs in COPD they do appear to reduce decline in lung function and exacerbations in patients with severe COPD. In patients with COPD and substantial but incomplete reversibility, they work by improving asthma outcomes	Oropharyngeal candidiasis, skin thinning, easy bruising, osteoporosis, cateracts (side-effects are dose- and duration dependent)
		AeroBec	BAMDI	50mcg, 100mcg			
		AeroBec Forte	BAMDI	250mcg			
		Asmabec Clickhaler	DPI	50mcg, 100mcg, 250mcg			
		Beclazone Easi-Breathe	MDI	50mcg, 100mcg			

Corticosteroids for COPD

Drug	Format	Trade names	Preparation	Strengths	Doses used in COPD	Comments	Side-effects
Beclometasone	Inhaled	Becodisks	DPI	100mcg, 200mcg, 400mcg	100-800mcg 2 times/d	While there is no clear mechanism for effectiveness of these drugs in COPD they do appear to reduce decline in lung function and exacerbations in patients with severe COPD. In patients with COPD and substantial but incomplete reversibility, they work by improving asthma outcomes	Oropharyngeal candidiasis, skin thinning, easy bruising, osteoporosis, cateracts (side-effects are dose- and duration dependent)
		Becotide	MDI	50mcg, 100mcg, 200mcg			
			MDI	250mcg			
		Becloforte	DPI	400mcg			
		Qvar	MDI	50mcg, 100mcg,			
			BAMDI	50mcg, 100mcg,			
Budesonide	Inhaled	Generic	DPI	200mcg, 400mcg	100-800mcg 2 times/d		
		Pulmicort	MDI	50mcg, 200mcg			
			Turbohaler	100mcg, 200mcg, 400mcg			
			Respules	250mcg/ml	1-2mg 2 times/d	Not recommended in COPD	
Fluticasone	Inhaled	Flixotide	MDI	25mcg, 50mcg, 125mcg, 250mcg	100-1000mcg 2 times/d		
			Accuhaler	50mcg, 100mcg, 250mcg, 500mcg			
			Diskhaler	50mcg, 100mcg, 250mcg, 500mcg			
			Nebules	250mcg/ml	500mcg-1mg 2 times/d	Not recommended in COPD	

Combined β$_2$-agonists and anticholinergics for COPD

Drug	Format	Trade names	Preparation	Strengths	Doses used in COPD	Comments	Side-effects
Salbutamol + Ipratropium	Inhaled	Combivent	MDI	100mcg Salbutamol + 20mcg Ipratropium	2 puffs 4 times/d	Because of differing mechanisms of actions the effects of these combinations, whether in one inhaler or two, appear to be additive. While this has been confirmed for short-acting bronchodilators it has not been formally studied for long-acting anticholinergics and β-agonists	Tachycardia, tremor, dry mouth
			Nebulizer Solution	2.5mg Salbutamol + 500mcg Ipratropium in 2.5 ml	1 vial 3-4 times/d		Tachycardia, tremor, dry mouth, brinary retention (rare), blurring of vision, acute glaucoma
Fenoterol + Ipratropium	Inhaled	Duovent	Nebulizer Solution	1.25mg Fenoterol + 500mcg Ipratropium in 4 ml	1 vial 3-4 times/d	Because of differing mechanisms of actions the effects of these combinations, whether in one inhaler or two, appear to be additive. While this has been confirmed for short-acting bronchodilators it has not been formally studied for long-acting anticholinergics and β-agonists	Tachycardia, tremor, dry mouth, urinary retention (rare), blurring of vision, acute glaucoma

Combined corticosteroids and long-acting β-agonists for COPD

Drug	Format	Trade names	Preparation	Strengths	Doses used in COPD	Comments	Side-effects
Budesonide + formoterol	Inhaled	Symbicort	Turbohaler	200mcg Budesonide + 6 mcg Eformoterol	2 puffs 2 times/d	These combine the effects and benefits of inhaled steroids and long-acting β-agonists. They are useful in those with severe disease to reduce exacerbations and protect against decline in quality of life (steroid effect) and to improve quality of life and symptoms (long-acting β-agonist effect)	Tremor, tachycardiia, hypokalaemia, oropharyngeal candidiasis, skin thinning, easy bruising, osteoporosis, cateracts (steroid side-effects are dose- and duration dependent)
				400mcg Budesonide + 12 mcg Eformoterol	1 puff 2 times/d		
Fluticasone + Salmeterol	Inhaled	Seretide	Accuhaler	500mcg Fluticasone + 50mcg Salmeterol	1 Inhaled 2 times/d	These combine the effects and benefits of inhaled steroids and long-acting β-agonists. They are useful in those with severe disease to reduce exacerbations and protect against decline in quality of life (steroid effect) and to improve quality of life and symptoms (long-acting β-agonist effect)	Tremor, tachycardiia, hypokalaemia, oropharyngeal candidiasis, skin thinning, easy bruising, osteoporosis, cateracts (steroid side-effects are dose- and duration dependent)

Quality indicators in the UK GP contract

Under the new general medical services contract, GPs can earn "indicator points" for the care of patients with asthma and COPD. Summary details are given below. Further information can be found at www.bma.org.uk/ap.nsf/Content/__HubGMScontractquality

Indicators for asthma	Points	Payment stages
Records		
ASTHMA 1. The practice can produce a register of patients with asthma, excluding patients with asthma who have been prescribed no asthma-related drugs in the last twelve months	7	
Initial management		
ASTHMA 2. The percentage of patients aged 8 and over diagnosed as having asthma from 1 April 2003 where the diagnosis has been confirmed by spirometry or peak flow measurement	15	25–70%
Ongoing management		
ASTHMA 3. The percentage of patients with asthma between age 14 and 19 in whom there is a record of smoking status in the previous 15 months	6	25–70%
ASTHMA 4. The percentage of patients aged 20 and over with asthma whose notes record smoking status in the past 15 months, except those who have never smoked where smoking status should be recorded at least once	6	25–70%
ASTHMA 5. The percentage of patients with asthma who smoke, and whose notes contain a record that smoking cessation advice or referral to a specialist service, if available, has been offered within the last 15 months	6	25–70%
ASTHMA 6. The percentage of patients with asthma who have had an asthma review in the last 15 months	20	25–70%
ASTHMA 7. The percentage of patients aged 16 and over with asthma who have had influenza immunisation in the preceding 1 September to 31 March	12	25–70%

Indicators for COPD	Points	Payment stages
Records		
COPD 1. The practice can produce a register of patients with COPD	5	
Initial diagnosis		
COPD 2. The percentage of patients in whom diagnosis has been confirmed by spirometry including reversibility testing for newly diagnosed patients with effect from 1 April 2003	5	25–90%
COPD 3. The percentage of all patients with COPD in whom diagnosis has been confirmed by spirometry including reversibility testing	5	25–90%
Ongoing management		
COPD 4. The percentage of patients with COPD in whom there is a record of smoking status in the previous 15 months	6	25–90%
COPD 5. The percentage of patients with COPD who smoke, whose notes contain a record that smoking cessation advice or referral to a specialist service, if available, has been offered in the past 15 months	6	25–90%
COPD 6. The percentage of patients with COPD with a record of FEV_1 in the previous 27 months	6	25–70%
COPD 7. The percentage of patients with COPD receiving inhaled treatment in whom there is a record that inhaler technique has been checked in the preceding 2 years	6	25–90%
COPD 8. The percentage of patients with COPD who have had influenza immunisation in the preceding 1 September to 31 March	6	25–85%

Abbreviations

BAI	Breath-activated inhaler
BDP	Beclomethasone dipropionate
BTS	British Thoracic Society
COPD	Chronic obstructive pulmonary disease
DPI	Dry powder inhaler
DV	Diurnal variability
FEV_1	Forced expiratory volume (amount of air forciby expelled in 1 second)
FVC	Forced vital capacity (total volume of air expelled from the lungs from maximium inhalation to maximum exhalation)
GORD	Gastro-oesophageal reflux disease
GPwSI	GPs with a special interest
ICS	Inhaled corticosteroid
IL	Interleukin
LABA	Long-acting ß_2-agonist
LTB_4	Leukotriene B_4
LTOT	Long-term oxygen therapy
LTRA	Leukotriene receptor antagonist
LVRS	Lung volume reduction surgery
MDI	Metered-dose inhaler
NNT	Number needed to treat
NRT	Nicotine replacement therapy
PAAP	Personalized asthma action plan
$PaCO_2$	Arterial partial pressure of carbon dioxide
PaO_2	Arterial partial pressure of oxygen
PCG	Primary care group
PCT	Primary care trust
PDE_4	Phosphodiesterase type 4
PEF	Peak expiratory flow
PEFR	Peak expiratory flow rate
RADS	Reactive airways dysfunction syndrome
RAST	Radioallergosorbent test
RSV	Respiratory syncytial virus
SABA	Short-acting ß_2-agonist
SIGN	Scottish intercollegiate guideline network
SpO_2	Arterial oxygen saturation
SWORD	Surveillance of work-related and occupational respiratory disease

Useful organizations

For the health professional

British Thoracic Society
The British Thoracic Society
17 Doughty Street
London
WC1N 2PY
Tel: 020 7831 8778
email: bts@brit-thoracic.org.uk
Website: www.brit-thoracic.org.uk

Cochrane Centre UK
Summertown Pavilion
Middleway
Oxford
OX2 7LG
Tel: 01865 516300
Website: www.cochrane.co.uk

Global Initiative for Chronic Obstructive Lung Disease (GOLD)
Romain Pauwels, M.D., Ph.D.
Email: shurd@prodigy.net
Website: www.goldcopd.com

General Practice Airways Group (GPIAG)
Website: www.gpiag.org

International Primary Care Respiratory Group
Website: www.theipcrg.org

National Respiratory Training Centre
The Athenaeum
10 Church Street
Warwick
CV34 4AB
Tel: 01926 493 313
Website: www.nartc.org.uk

Oasys and Occupational Asthma
http://www.occupationalasthma.com

National Heart, Lung and Blood Institute
NHLBI Health Information Center
PO Box 30105
Bethesda, MD 20824-0105, USA
Tel: 001 301 592 8573
Email: nhlbiinfo@rover.nhlbi.nih.gov
Website: www.nhlbi.nih.gov/

Respiratory Education and Training Centres
University Hospital Aintree
Lower Lane
Liverpool
L9 7AL
Tel: 0151 5292598
Website: www.respiratoryetc.com

Royal Pharmaceutical Society of Great Britain
1 Lambeth High Street
London
SE1 7JN
Tel: 020 7735 9141
Email: enquiries@rpsgb.org.uk
Website: www.rpsgb.org.uk

Scottish Intercollegiate Guidelines Network (SIGN)
9 Queen Street,
Edinburgh
EH2 1JQ
Tel: 0131-225 7324
Website: www.sign.ac.uk

World Health Organisation Regional Office for Europe
8, Scherfigsvej
DK-2100 Copenhagen 0
Denmark
Tel: +45 39 171 717
E-mail: postmaster@euro.who.int
Website: www.who/int/en

For the patient

Age Concern England
Astral House
1268 London Road
London
SW16 4ER
Tel: 0800 009966
Website: www.ageconcern.org.uk

Age Concern Scotland
Leonard Small House
113 Rose Street
Edinburgh
EH2 3DT
Tel: 0800 00 99 66
Website: ageconcernscotland.org.uk

Benefits Agency helpline
Tel: 0800 882 200

Breathe Easy Groups
See British Lung Foundation for contact information
Website: www.lunguk.org/breathe.asp

British Lung Foundation
78 Hatton Garden
London
EC1N 8 LD
Tel: 020 7831 5831
Website: www.lunguk.org

National Asthma Campaign
Providence House
Providence Place
London
N1 0NT
Tel: 020 7226 2260
Website: www.asthma.org.uk

NHS Smoking Helpline
Tel: 0800 169 0169

References

1. British Thoracic Society. *The Burden of Lung Disease*. London: British Thoracic Society, 2001
2. National Asthma Audit 1999/2000. Summary. Factsheet 18. London: National Asthma Campaign, 1999
3. Upton MN *et al*. Intergenerational 20-year trends in the prevalence of asthma and hayfever in adults: the Midspan family study surveys of parents and offspring. *BMJ* 2000;**321**:88–92
4. Omran M, Russell G. Continuing increase in respiratory symptoms and atopy in Aberdeen schoolchildren. *BMJ* 1996;**312**:34
5. Murray CJL, Lopez AD (eds). *The Global Burden of Disease: a comprehensive assessment of mortality and disability from diseases, injuries and risk factors in 1990 and projected to 2020.* Cambridge, MA: Havard School of Public Health on behalf of the World Health Organization and the World Bank (Global Burden of Disease and Injury Series, Vol. I), 1996
6. Lundback B *et al*. Not 15 but 50% of smokers develop COPD? – Report from the Obstructive Lung Disease in Northern Sweden Studies. *Respir Med* 2003;**97**:115–22
7. Price D, Freeman D. The BREATH (Breathlessness Research, Expectations and Treatment Hopes) study: findings of a pilot study in four countries. *Prim Care Resp J* 2002;**11**:S12–S14
8. Tirimanna PR, van Schayck CP, den Otter JJ et al. Prevalence of asthma and COPD in general practice in 1992: has it changed since 1977? *Br J Gen Pract* 1996;**46**:277–81
9. Lindstrom M, Jonsson E, Larsson K, Lundback B. Underdiagnosis of obstructive lung disease in northern Sweden. *Int J Tuber Lung Dis* 2002;**6**:78–84
10. Charlton I, Charlton G, Broomfield J *et al*. Audit of the effect of a nurse run asthma clinic on workload and patient morbidity in a general practice. *Br J Gen Pract* 1991;**41**:227–31
11. Ostrem A, Freeman D, Foster J *et al*. A pilot survey undertaken by the IPCRG of international delivery of care for COPD. *Prim Care Resp J* 2002;**11**:67 [Abstract]
12. Drummond N, Abdalla M, Buckingham J K *et al*. Integrated care for asthma: a clinical, social, and economic evaluation. *BMJ* 1994;**308**:559–64
13. Bourke SJ, Brewis RAL. Respiratory Medicine. Oxford: Blackwell Science, 1988
14. British Thoracic Society (BTS) and Scottish Intercollegiate Guidelines Network (SIGN). British guideline on the management of asthma. *Thorax* 2003;**58 (Suppl I)**:1–94
15. National Institutes of Health international consensus report on the diagnosis and treatment of asthma. National Heart, Lung and Blood Institute, National Institutes of Health, Bethesda, Maryland 20892. Publication no. 92–3091. *Eur Respir J* 1992;**5**:601–41
16. Schlecht H, Schwenker G. Uber die Beziehungen der Eosinophilie zur Anaphylaxie. *Ditsch Arch Klin Med* 1912;**108**:405–28
17. Sears MR. Epidemiology. In: Barnes PJ, Rodger IW, Thomson NC (eds). *Asthma: basic mechanisms and clinical management*, 2nd edn. San Diego: Academic Press, p119,1992
18. Burney PG, Chinn S, Rona RJ. Has the prevalence of asthma increased in children? Evidence from the national study of health and growth 1973–86. *BMJ* 1990;**300**:1306–10
19. Omran M, Russell G. Continuing increase in respiratory symptoms and atopy in Aberdeen schoolchildren. *BMJ* 1996;**312**:34
20. Sears MR. Descriptive epidemiology of asthma. *Lancet* 1997;**350**:14
21. Pearce N, Weiland S, Keil U *et al*. Self-reported prevalence of asthma symptoms in children in Australia, England, Germany and New Zealand: an international comparison using the ISAAC protocol. *Eur Respir J* 1993;**6**:1455–61
22. Oswald H, Phelan PD, Lanigan A *et al*. Outcome of childhood asthma in mid-adult life. *BMJ* 1994;**309**:95–6
23. Jenkins MA, Hopper JL, Bowes G *et al*. Factors in childhood as predictors of asthma in adult life. *BMJ* 1994;**309**:90–3
24. Strachan DP, Butland BK, Anderson HR. Incidence and prognosis of asthma and wheezing illness from early childhood to age 33 in a national British cohort. *BMJ* 1996;**312**:1195–6
25. Martinez FD, Wright AL, Taussig LM *et al*. Asthma and wheezing in the first six years of life. The Group Health Associates. *N Engl J Med* 1995;**332**:133–8
26. Dubois P, Degrave E, Vandenplas O. Asthma and airway hyperresponsiveness among Belgian conscripts 1978–91. *Thorax* 1998;**53**:101–5

127

27. Haahtela T, Lindholm H, Bjorksten F *et al.* Prevalence of asthma in Finnish young men. *BMJ* 1990;**301**:266–8

28. Upton MN, McConnachie A, McSharry C *et al.* Intergenerational 20 year trends in the prevalence of asthma and hayfever in adults: the Midspan family study surveys of parents and offspring. *BMJ* 2000;**321**:88–92

29. Sears, MR, Willan A, Herbison GP *et al.* Associations between atopy, hyperresponsiveness and persistence of childhood asthma. *Eur Respir J* 1997;**10**:162S

30. Spork R, Chapman MD, Platts-Mills TAE. House dust mite exposure as a cause of asthma. *Clin Exper Allergy* 1992;**22**:896–906

31. Martinez FD, Wright AL, Taussig LM *et al.* Asthma and wheezing in the first six years of life. *N Engl J Med* 1995;**32**:133–8

32. Fleming DM, Sunderland R, Cross KW *et al.* Declining incidence of episodes of asthma: a study of trends in new episodes presenting to general practitioners in the period 1989–98. *Thorax* 2000;**55**:657–61

33. Baldwin DR, Ormerod LP, Mackay AD, Stableforth DE. Change in hospital management of acute severe asthma by general and thoracic physicians in Birmingham and Manchester during 1978 and 1985. *Thorax* 1990;**45**:130–5

34. Pearce N, Pekkanen J, Beasley R. How much asthma is really attributable to atopy? *Thorax* 1999;**54**:268–72

35. Los H, Koppelman G, Postma D. The importance of genetic influences in asthma. *Eur Respir J* 1999;**14**:1210–27

36. MMWR. Current trends in asthma in the United States 1982–1992. *Morbid Mortal Wkly Rep* 1995;**43**:952–5

37. Weiss KB, Wagener DK. Changing patterns of asthma mortality: identifying target populations at high risk. *J Am Med Assoc* 1990;**264**:1683–7

38. Weiss KB, Wagener DK. Geographic variations in US asthma mortality: small-area analyses of excess mortality, 1981–1985. *Am J Epidemio*l 1990;**132**(Suppl. 1): S107–S115

39. Sporik R, Holgate ST, Platts-Mills TA, Cogswell JJ. Exposure to house-dust mite allergen (Der p I) and the development of asthma in childhood. A prospective study. *N Engl J Med* 1990;**323**(8):502–7

40. Samet JM, Lambert WE. Epidemiologic approaches for assessing health risks from complex mixtures in indoor air. *Environ. Health Perspectives* 1991;**95**:71–74

41. Speizer FE. Asthma and persistent wheeze in the Harvard six cities study. *Chest* 1990;**98**:191S–195S

42. Folkerts G, Busse W, Nijkamp F *et al.* State of the art: virus-induced airway hyperresponsiveness and asthma. *Am J Respir Crit Care Med* 1998 **157**:1708–20

43. Chan-Yeung M, Malo JL. Occupational asthma. N *Engl J Med* 1995;**333**(2):107–12

44. Park JH, Gold DR, Spiegelman DL *et al.* House dust endotoxin and wheeze in the first year of life. *Am J Respir Crit Care Med* 2001;**163**(2):322–28

45. Gereda J, Leung D, Thatayatikom A *et al.*Relation between house-dust endotoxin exposure, type 1 T-cell development, and allergen sensitization in infants at high risk of asthma. *Lancet* 2000;**355**:1680–3

46. Rylander R, Haglind P, Lundholm M. Endotoxin in cotton dust and respiratory function decrement among cotton workers in an experimental cardroom. *Am Rev Respir Dis* 1985;**131**:209–13

47. Donham K, Haglind P, Peterson Y. Environmental and health studies of farm workers in Swedish swine confinement buildings. *Br J Ind Med* 1989;**46**:31–7

48. Lichtenstein P, Svatengren M. Genes, environments, and sex: factors of importance in atopic diseases in 79-year-old Swedish twins. *Allergy* 1997;**52**:1079–86

49. Khoury MJ, Beaty TH, Cohen BH. Fundamentals of genetic epidemiology. In: Khoury MJ, Beaty TH, Cohen BH (eds). *Genetic Approaches to Familial Aggregation. I. Analysis of Heritability* . Oxford: Oxford University Press, pp. 200–32, 1993

50. Edfors-Lubs ML. Allergy in 7000 twin pairs. *Acta Allergol* 1971;**26**:249–85

51. Chan-Yeung M, Manfreda J, Dimich-Ward H. A randomized controlled study on the effectiveness of a multifaceted intervention program in the primary prevention of asthma in high-risk infants. *Arch Pediatr Adolesc Med* 2000;**154**:657–63

52. Los H, Koppelman G, Postma D. The importance of genetic influences in asthma. *Eur Respir J* 1999;**14**:1210–27

53. Maddox L,Schwartz DA. The pathophysiology of asthma. *Ann Rev Med* 2002;**53**:477–98

54. Van Eerdewegh P, Little RD *et al.* Association of the ADAM33 gene with asthma and bronchial hyperresponsiveness. *Nature* 2002; **418**(6896):426–30

55. Holgate ST. Asthma genetics: waiting to exhale. *Nat Genet* 1997;**15**:227–9

56. Martinez FD, Holt PG. Role of microbial burden in aetiology of allergy and asthma. *Lancet* 1999;**354**(suppl II):12–5

57. Busse WW, Lemanske RF. Asthma. *N Engl J Med* 2001;**344**(5):350–62

58. von Mutius E *et al.* Exposure to endotoxin or other bacterial components might protect against the development of atopy. *Clin Exper Allergy* 2000;**30**:1230–4
59. Lapa e Silva JR, Possebon da Silva MD, Lefort J *et al.* Endotoxins, asthma, and allergic immune responses. *Toxicology* 2000;**152**:31–5
60. Simpson A, Custovic A. Early pet exposure: friend or foe? *Curr Opin Allergy Clin Immunol* 2003;**3(1)**:7–14
61. Riedler J, Eder W, Oberfield G *et al.* Austrian children living on a farm have less hayfever, asthma and allergic sensitization. *Clin Exper Allergy* 2000;**30**:194–200
62. Lemanske RF. Issues in understanding pediatric asthma: epidemiology and genetics. *J Allergy Clin Immunol* 2002; **109(6 Suppl)**:S521–24
63. Wafula EM, Limbe MS, Onyango FE *et al.* Effects of passive smoking and breastfeeding on childhood bronchial asthma. *East Afr Med J* 1999;**76**:606–9
64. Romieu I, Werneck G, Velasco SR *et al.* Breastfeeding and asthma among Brazilian children. *J Asthma* 2000;**37**: 575–83
65. Wright AL, Holberg CJ, Taussig LM *et al.* Factors influencing the relation of infant feeding to asthma and recurrent wheeze in childhood. *Thorax* 2001;**56**:192–7
66. Rusconi F, Galassi C, Corbo GM *et al*, for the SIDRIA collaborative group. Risk factors for early, persistent, and late-onset wheezing in young children. *Am J Respir Crit Care Med* 1999;**160**:1617–22
67. Sears MR, Greene JM, Willan AR *et al.* Long-term relation between breastfeeding and development of atopy and asthma in children and young adults: a longitudinal study. *Lancet* 2002;**360**:901–7
68. Sigurs N. Epidemiologic and clinical evidence of a respiratory syncytial virus-reactive airway disease link. *Am J Respir Crit Care Med* 2001;**163**:S2–S6
69. Gern J, Lemanske RF Jr, Busse W. Early life origins of asthma. *J Clin Invest* 1999;**104(7)**:837–43
70. Christiansen S. Day care, siblings, and asthma — please, sneeze on my child. *N Engl J Med* 2000;**343(8)**:574–75
71. Holgate ST. The inflammation-repair cycle in asthma: the pivotal role of the airway epithelium. In Holgate S T, Boushey H A, Fabbri L M (eds). *Difficult Asthma.* London: Martin Dunitz, pp. 13–21, 1999
72. Castro M, Chaplin D, Walter M *et al.* Could asthma be worsened by stimulating the T-helper type 1 immune response? *Am J Respir Cell Mol Biol* 2000;**22**:143–6
73. Hansen G, Berry G, DeKruyff RH *et al.* Allergen-specific Th1 cells fail to counterbalance T$_{H}$2 cell-induced airway hyperreactivity but cause severe airway inflammation. *J Clin Invest* 1999;**103**:175–83
74. Koppleman GH, Los H, Postma DS. Genetic and environment in asthma: the answer of twin studies. *Eur Resp J* 1999;**13 (1)**:2–4
75. Bousquet J, Jeffery P, Busse W *et al.* Asthma: from bronchoconstriction to airways inflammation and remodeling. *Am J Respir Crit Care Med* 2000;**161**:1720–45
76. Chung KF, Adcock IM. Pathophysiological mechanisms of asthma. Application of cell and molecular biology techniques. *Mol Biotech* 2001;**18(3)**:213–32
77. Busse WW, Lemanske RF. Asthma. *N Engl J Med* 2001;**344(5)**:350–62
78. Rothenberg ME. Eosinophilia. *N Engl J Med* 1998;**338(22)**:1592–600
79. Holt PG, Macaubas C, Stumbles PA *et al.* The role of allergy in the development of asthma. *Nature* 1999;**402(6760 Suppl)**:B12–17
80. Holgate ST. Asthma therapy in the new millenium. *Allergology Internat* 2000;**49**: 231–6
81. Hanazawa T, Kharitonov SA, Barnes PJ. Increased nitrotyrosine in exhaled breath condensate of patients with asthma. *Am J Respir Crit Care Med* 2000;**162**:1273–6
82. Elias J, Zhum A, Chupp G *et al.* Airway remodeling in asthma. *J Clin Invest* 1999;**104(8)**:1001–6
83. Dilworth JP, Baldwin DR. Respiratory Medicine Specialist Handbook. London and New York: Martin Dunitz, 2002
84. Chung F, Fabbri LM. Asthma. European Respiratory Monograph. European Respiratory Society Journals ltd, 2003
85. Banks DE, Wang ML. Occupational asthma "the big picture". *Occupat Asthma* 2000;**15**:335–58
86. Ross DJ. Ten years of the SWORD project. *Clin Exper Allergy* 1999;**29**:750–3
87. Cartier A. Definition of occupational asthma. *Eur Respir J* 1994;**7**:153–60
88. Paggario PL, Vagaggini Bm Bacci E *et al.* Prognosis of occupational asthma. *Eur Resp J* 1994;**7**:761–7
89. Chan-Yeung M, Maclean L, Paggiario PL. Follow-up study of 232 patients with occupational asthma caused by western red cedar (*Thuja plicata*). *J Allergy Clin Immunol* 1987;**79**:792–6

90. Cartier A, Bernstein IL, Burge PS *et al.* Guidelines for bronchoprovocation on the investigation of occupational asthma. Report of the Subcommittee on Bronchoprovocation for Occupational Asthma. *J Allergy Clin Immunol* 1989; **84**:823–9

91. Paggario PL, Vagaggini B, Bacci E *et al.* Prognosis of occupational asthma. *Eur Resp J* 1994;7:761–7

92. Gannon PF, Weir DC, Robertson AS *et al.* Health, employment and financial outcomes in workers with occupational asthma. *Br J Ind Med* 1993;**50**:91–66

93. Thomas M, McKinley RK, Freeman E, Foy C. Prevalence of dysfunctional breathing in patients treated for asthma in primary care: cross sectional survey. *BMJ* 2001;322:1098–100

94. Thomas M, McKinley RK, Freeman E *et al.* Breathing retraining for dysfunctional breathing in asthma: a randomized controlled trial. *Thorax.* 2003;**58**:110–5

95. Price D, Ryan D, Pearce L *et al.* The AIR study: asthma in real life. *Asthma J* 1999;4:74–8

96. Price D, Ryan D, Pearce L *et al.* The burden of paediatric asthma is higher than health professionals think: results from the Asthma In Real Life (AIR) study. *Prim Care Respir J* 2002;**11(2)**:30–1

97. Pinnock H, Bawden R, Proctor S *et al.* Accessibility, acceptability, and effectiveness in primary care of routine telephone review of asthma: pragmatic, randomized controlled trial. *BMJ* 2003;**326**:477–9

98. Laitinen LA, Laitinen A, Haahtela T. A comparative study of the effects of an inhaled corticosteroid, budesonide, and a beta$_2$-agonist, terbutaline, on airway inflammation in newly diagnosed asthma: a randomized, double-blind, parallel-group controlled trial. *J Allergy Clin Immunol* 1992;**90(1)**:32–42

99. Hanania NA, Chapman KR, Kesten S. Adverse Effects of Inhaled Corticosteroids. *Am J Med* 1994;**98**:196–207

100. The Childhood Asthma Management Program Research Group. Long-term effects of budesonide or nedocromil in children with asthma. *N Engl J Med* 2000;**343**: 1054–63

101. Drake AJ, Howells RJ, Shield JPH, et al. Symptomatic adrenal insufficiency presenting with hypoglycaemia in children with asthma receiving high dose inhaled fluticasone propionate. *BMJ* 2002;**324**:1081–3

102. Price DB, Hernandez D, Magyar P *et al* for the Clinical Outcomes with Montelukast as a Partner Agent to Corticosteroid Therapy (COMPACT) International Study Group. Randomized controlled trial of montelukast plus inhaled budesonide versus double dose inhaled budesonide in adult patients with asthma *Thorax* 2003;**58**:211–6

103. Vaquerizo MJ, Casan P, Castillo J *et al.* Effect of montelukast added to inhaled budesonide on control of mild to moderate asthma. *Thorax* 2003;**58**:204–10

104. Bourke SJ, Brewis RAL. *Respiratory Medicine,* 5th edn. Oxford: Blackwell Science, 1988

105. Lahdensuo A, Muittari A. Bronchodilator effects of a fenoterol metered dose inhaler and fenoterol powder in asthmatics with poor inhaler. *Eur J Respir Dis* 1986;**68**:332–5

106. Kamps AW, Van Ewijk B, Roorda RJ *et al.* Poor inhalation technique even after inhalation instructions, in children with *Pediatric Pulmonol* 2000;**29**:3942

107. Newman SP. Improvement of drug delivery with a breath actuated pressurized aerosol for patients with poor inhaler *Thorax* 1991;**46**:712–26

108. Brocklebank D, Wright J, Cates C. Systematic review of clinical effectiveness of pressurized metered dose inhalers versus other hand held inhaler devices for delivering corticosteroids in asthma. *BMJ* 2001;**323**:901–11

109. Ram F, Wright J, Brocklebank D *et al.* Systematic review of clinical effectiveness of pressurized metered dose inhalers versus other hand held inhaler devices for delivering B2 agonists bronchodilators in asthma. *BMJ* 2001;**323**:896–900

110. Price D, Thomas M, Mitchell G, et al. Improvement of asthma control wit a breath actuated pressurized metred dose inhaler (BAI):a prescribing claims study of 5556 patients using a traditional pressurized metred dose inhaler (MDI) or a breath-actuated device. *Resp Med* 2003;**97**:12–9

111. Bisgaard H. Delivery of inhaled medication to children. *J Asthma* 1997;**34**:443–67

112. Anhøj J, Bisgaard H, Lipworth BJ. Effect of electrostatic charge in plastic spacers on the lung delivery of HFA-salbutamol in children. *Br J Clin Pharmacol* 1999;**47**:333–6

113. Wildhaber JH, Janssens HM, Pierart F *et al.* High-percentage lung delivery in children from detergent-treated spacers. *Pediatr Pulmonol* 2000;**29**:389–93

114. Cotterell EM, Gazarian M, Henry RL, *et al.* Child and parent satisfaction with the use of spacer devices in acute asthma. *J Paediatr Child Health* 2002;**38(6)**:604–7

115. British Thoracic Society. Current best practice for nebuliser treatment. *Thorax* 1997;**52(Suppl 2)**:S1–S106

116. Lehrer PM, Hochron SM, Mayne T *et al.* Relationship between changes in EMG and respiratory sinus arrhythmia in a study of relaxation therapy for asthma. *Appl Psychophysiol Biofeedback* 1997;**22(3)**:183–91

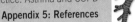

117. Garden GM, Ayres JG. Psychiatric and social aspects of brittle asthma. *Thorax* 1993 **48(5)**:501–5

118. Miles JF, Garden GM, Tunnicliffe WS *et al.* Psychological morbidity and coping skills in patients with brittle and non-brittle asthma: a case-control study. *Clin Exper Allergy* 1997;**27(10)**:1151–9

119. Bosley CM, Corden ZM, Cochrane GM. Psychosocial factors and asthma. *Respir Med* 1996;**90**:453–7

120. Kotses H, Bernstein IL, Bernstein DI. A self-management program for adult asthma. Part 1: Development and evaluation. *J Allergy Clin Immunol*, 1995;**95(2)**: 529–40

121. Bailey WC, Richards JM, Brooks C *et al.* A randomized trial to improve self-management practices of adults with asthma. *Arch Intern Med* 1990;**150**:1664–8

122. Henry M, De Rivera G, Gonzales-Martin IJ *et al* Improvement of respiratory function in chronic asthmatic patients with autogenic therapy. *J Psychomatic Res* 1993;**37(3)**:265–70

123. Flemming S, Shuldham C, Churchill R *et al.* Psychotherapeutic interventions for adults with asthma (Cochrane Review). In: *The Cochrane Library*, Issue 4, (2002). Oxford: Update Software

124. Devine EC. Meta-analysis of the effects of psychoeducational care in adults with asthma. *Res Nursing Health* 1996;**19**:367–76

125. Pagliari C, Shuldham C, Fleming S *et al.* Psychotherapeutic interventions for children with asthma (Cochrane Review). In: *The Cochrane Library*, Issue 4, (2002). Oxford: Update Software

126. Gallefoss F, Bakke PS. Impact of patient education and self-management on morbidity in asthmatics and patients with chronic obstructive pulmonary disease. *Respir Med* 2000;**94**:279–87

127. Lahdensuo A, Haahtela T, Herrala J *et al.* Randomized comparison of guided self management and traditional treatment of asthma over one year *BMJ* 1996;**312**:748–52

128. Toelle BG, Ram FSF. Written individualized management plans for asthma in children and adults. [Systematic Review] Cochrane Airways Group. *Cochrane Database of Systematic Reviews* 2003;1

129. Gibson PG, Powell H, Coughlan J, *et al.* Self-management education andregular practitioner review for adults with asthma. [Systematic Review] *Cochrane Database of Systematic Reviews* 2003;1

130. Pinnock HJ, Johnson A, Young P, Martin N. Are doctors still failing to assess and treat asthma attacks? An audit of the management of acute attacks in a Health District. *Respir Med* 1999;93: 397–401

131. Neville RG, Clark RC, Hoskins G, Smith B for GPIAG. National asthma attack audit 1991–2. *BMJ* 1993;**306**: 559–62

132. British Thoracic Association. Death from asthma in two regions of England. *BMJ* 1982;**285**:1251–5

133. Lindberg M, Ahlner J, Moller M *et al.* Asthma nurse practice — a resource-effective approach to asthma management. *Respir Med* 1999;**93**:584–8

134. Heard AR, Richards IJ, Alpers JH *et al.* Randomised controlled trial of general practice-based asthma clinics. *Med J Aust* 1999;**171**:68–71

135. Drummond N, Abdalla M, Buckingham J K *et al.* for Grampian Asthma Study of Integrated Care (GRASSIC). Integrated care for asthma: a clinical, social, and economic evaluation. *BMJ* 1994;**308**:559–64

136. Department of Health. *The NHS Plan: A Plan for Investment, A Plan for Reform* (2002). London: The Stationery Office

137. Williams S, Ryan D, Price D, *et al.* General practitioners with a special clinical interest: a model for improving respiratory disease management. *Br J Gen Pract* 2002;**52**:838–43

138. Royal College of General Practitioners. Clinical governance: practical advice for primary care in England and Wales. [College Viewpoint] London: RCGP, 1999

139. British Thoracic Society. *The Burden of Lung Disease*. Factsheet 20001/4. London: BTS, 2001

140. Guest JF. The annual cost of chronic obstructive pulmonary disease to the UK's National Health Service. *Dis Manag Health Outcomes* 1999;**5(2)**:93–100

141. Lopez AD, Murray CC. The global burden of disease, 1990–2020. *Nat Med* 1998;**4(11)**:1241–3

142. National Heart, Lung and Blood Institute. Global Strategy for the Diagnosis, Management and Prevention of Chronic Obstructive Pulmonary Disease. NHLBI, 2001

143. Barnes PJ. *Managing Chronic Obstructive Pulmonary Disease.* London: Science Press, 1999

144. Crockett A. Managing Chronic Obstructive Pulmonary Disease in Primary Care. Oxford: Blackwell Science, 2000

145. COPD Guidelines Group of the Standards of Care Committee of the BTS. BTS guidelines for the management of chronic obstructive pulmonary disease. *Thorax* 1997;**52(Suppl 5)**:S1–S28

146. Dickinson JA, Meaker M, Searle M *et al.* Screening in older patients for chronic obstructive airways disease in a semi-rural practice. *Thorax* 1999;**54**:501–5

147. Renwick DS, Conolly MJ. Prevalence and treatment of chronic airways obstruction in adults over the age of 45. *Thorax* 1996;**51**:164–8

148. Halpin DMG. *COPD.* London: Harcourt Brace, 2001

149. Anderson RH, Esmail A, Hollowell J, *et al.* Epidemiologically based needs assessment: lower respiratory disease. London: HMSO, 1994

150. Calverley PJ. *Chronic Obstructive Pulmonary Disease (COPD) The Lung Report.* London: British Lung Foundation, 1997

151. Osman IM, Godden DJ, Friend JA *et al.* Quality of life and hospital re-admission in patients with chronic obstructive pulmonary disease. *Thorax,* 1997;**52**:67–71

152. British Thoracic Society. The Burden of Lung Disease [online]. Available from: http://www.brit-thoracic.org.uk/pdf/BTSpages.pdf [Accessed 25th March 2003].

153. Turato G, Zuin R, Baroldo S *et al.* Lung pathology in chronic obstrucitve pulmonary disease. Available from http://www.copdprofessional.org/literature/big_articles/suetta.html. [Accessed February 2003]

154. Godden DJ, Douglas A. *Clinicians Manual on Chronic Obstructive Pulmonary Disease.* London: Science Press, 2002

155. Van Schayck CP, Chavannes NH. Detection of asthma and chronic obstructive pulmonary disease in primary care. *Eur Respir J* 2003;**21(Suppl 39)**:16s–22s

156. Celli BR. The importance of spirometry in COPD and asthma. *Chest* 2000;**117**:15s–19s

157. Godden DJ, Douglas A. Clinician's Manual on Chronic Obstructive Pulmonary Disease. London: Science Press, 2000

158. GOLD Workshop Panel. *Global Strategy for the Diagnosis, Management, and Prevention of Chronic Obstructive Pulmonary Disease: NHLBI/ WHO Workshop Report* (2003) [online]. Available at: http://www.goldcopd.com [Accessed 25th March 2003]

159. Van Schyack CP, Loozen JM, Wagena E *et al.* Detecting patients at a high risk of developing chronic obstructive pulmonary disease in general practice: cross-sectional case finding study. *BMJ* 2002;**324(7350)**:1370

160. Pauwels RA. National and International Guidelines for COPD: The need for evidence. *Chest* 2000;**117**:20s–22s

161. O'Donnell DE. Assessment of bronchodilator efficacy in symptomatic COPD: Is spirometry useful? *Chest* 2000;**117**:42s–47s

162. Calverley PJ, Sondhi S. The burden of obstructive lung disease in the UK — COPD and asthma. *Thorax* 1998;**53(Suppl 4)**:A83

163. Fletcher C, Peto R. The natural history of chronic airflow obstruction. *BMJ* 1977;**1**:1645–8

164. Anthonisen NR, Connett JE, Kiley JP *et al.* Effects of smoking intervention and the use of as inhaled anticholinergic bronchodilator on the rate of decline of FEV_1: The Lung Health Study *JAMA* 1994;**16(272)**:1497–505

165. Kanner RE, Connett JE, Williams DE, Buist AS. Effects of randomized assignment to a smoking cezsation intervention and changes in smoking habits in smokers with early chronic obstructive pulmonary disease: The Lung Health Study. *Am J Med* 1999;**106(4)**:410–6

166. Coleman T, Wilson A. Anti-smoking advice from general practitioners: Is a population-based approach to advice-giving feasible? *Br J General Practice* 2000;**50**:1001–4

167. Silagy C, Stead LF. Physician advice for smoking cessation. (Cochrane Review) *The Cochrane Library,* Issue 4, (2002). Oxford: Update Software

168. Lancaster T, Stead LF. Individual behavioural counselling for smoking ceszation (Cochrane Review). *The Cochrane Library,* Issue 4 (2002) Oxford: Update Software

169. Department of Health. *Smoking Kills: A White Paper on Tobacco.* London: HMSO, 1998

170. Gourlay SG, McNeil JJ. Antismoking products. *Med J Austral* 1990;**153**:699–707

171. Henningfield JE, Fant RV, Gopalan L. Non-nicotine medications for smoking cessation. *J Respir Dis* 1998;**19(Suppl 8)**:S33–S42

172. Silagy C, Mant D, Fowler G, Lancaster T. Nicotine replacement therapy for smoking ceszation (Cochrane Review). *The Cochrane Library,* Issue 4, 2001, Oxford: Update Software

173. Abelin T, Buehler A, Muller P *et al.* Controlled trial of transdermal nicotine patch in tobacco withdrawal. *Lancet* 1989;**1**:7–10

174. Killen JD, Fortmann SP, Newman B, Varady A. Evaluation of a treatment approach combining nicotine gum with self-guided behavioural treatments for smoking relapse prevention. *J Consult Clin Psychol* 1990;**58**:85–92

175. Wallstrom M, Nilsson F, Hirsch JM. A randomized, double-blind, placebo-controlled clinical evaluation of a nicotune sublingual tablet in smoking cessation. *Addiction* 2000;**95(8)**:1161–71

176. Hughes JR, Stead LF, Lancaster T. Antidepressants for smoking cessation (Cochrane Review). *The Cochrane Library* Issue 4, 2002 Oxford: Update Software

177. Hurt RD, Sachs DP, Glover ED *et al.* A comparison of sustained release bupropion and placebo for smoking cessation. *N Eng J Med* 1997;**337**:1195–202

178. Silagy C, Lancaster T, Stead L, *et al.* Nicotine replacement therapy for smoking cessation. Cochrane Database Systematic Review. 2001;3:CD000146.

179. Parayil R, Jones N, Chavannes A, *et al.* A108 [Poster: C75] The meaning of COPD and its exacerbations to patients in the UK, Denmark and the Netherlands. ATS, 2003

180. Calverley PJ. *Chronic Obstructive Pulmonary Disease: The Key Facts.* London: British Lung Foundation, 1998

181. Kanner RE. Early intervention in chronic obstructive pulmonary disease: A review of the Lung Health Study results. *Med Clin North Am* 1996;**80**:523–47

182. Jones PW, Bosh TK. Quality of life changes in COPD patients treated with salmeterol. *Am J Crit Care Med* 2001;**163(5)**:1087–1092

183. Appleton S, Smith B, Veale A, Bara A. Long-acting beta $_2$-agonists for chronic obstructive pulmonary disease. *Cochrane Database Syst Rev* 2000;**(3)**:754–6

184. Brusasco V, Hodder R, Miravitiles M et al. Health outcomes following treatment for six months with once daily tiotropium compared with twice daily salmeterol in patients with COPD. Thorax 2003;58:399–404185. Vincken W, van Noord JA, Bateman ED *et al.* Improved health outcomes in patients with COPD during 1 year's treatment with tiotropium. *Eur Respir J* 2002;**19**:209–16

186. Casaburi R, Mahler DA, Jones PW *et al.* A long- term evaluation of once-daily inhaled tiotropioum in chronic obstructive pulmonary disease. *Eur Respir J* 2002;**19**:217–24

187. Barnes PJ. New therapies for chronic obstructive pulmonary disease. *Thorax* 1998;**52(2)**:137–47

188. Burge PS, Calverley PM, Jones PW *et al.* Randomised, double blind, placebo controlled study of fluticasone propionate in patients with moderate to severe chronic obstructive pulmonary disease: The Isolde trial. *BMJ* 2000;**320(7245)**:1279–303

189. The Lung Health Study Research Group. Effect of inhaled triacinolone on the decline in pulmonary function in chronic obstructive pulmonary disease. *N Engl J Med* 2000;**343**:1902–9

190. COMBIVENT Inhalation Aerosol Study Group, In chronic obstructive pulmonary disease, a combination of ipratropium and albuterol is more effective than either agent alone. An 85-day mutlicenter trial. *Chest* 1994;**105(5)**:1411–9

191. Multicenter Study Group. Long term oral acetylcysteine in chronic bronchitis:a double-blind controlled study. *Eur J Respir Dis* 1980;**111(Suppl)**:93–108

192. Gerrits CMJM, Herings RMC, Leufkens HGM , Lammers J-WJ. N-acetylcysteine reduces the risk of re-hospitalisation among patients with chronic obstructive pulmonary disease. *Eur Resp J* 2003;**21**:795-798

193. Foxwell AR, Cripps AWC. Haemophilus influenzae oral vaccination for preventing acute exacerbations of chronic bronchitis. (Cochrane Review). *The Cochrane Library*, Issue 4 2000. Oxford: Update Software

194. Gorse GJ, Otto EE, Daughaday CC *et al.* Influenza virus vaccination of patients with chronic lung disease. *Chest* 1997;**112(5)**:1221–33

195. Hak E, van Essen GA, Buskens E *et al.* Is immunising all patients with chronic lung disease in the community against influenza cost effective? Evidence from a general practice-based clinical prospective cohort study in Utrecht, The Netherlands. *J Epidemiol Comm Health* 1998;**52(2)**:120–5

196. Nichol KL, Baken L, Wuorenma J, Nelson A. The health and economic benefits associated with pneumococcal vaccination of elderly persons with chronic lung disease. *Arch Intern Med* 1999;**159(20)**:2437–42

197. Bent S, Saint S, Vittinghoff E, Grady D. Antibiotics in acute bronchitis: a meta-analysis. *Am J Med* 1990;**107(1)**:62–67

198. Barnes PJ. Chronic obstructive pulmonary disease. *New Engl J Med* 2000;**343**:269–80

199. Ram FSF. Regular inhaled short acting B2 agonists for the management of stable chronic obstructive pumonary disease: Cochrane systematic review and meta-analysis. *Thorax* 2003;**58**:580-4

133

200. Newhouse M, Dolovich M. Aerosol therapy: nebulizer vs metered dose inhaler. *Chest* 1987;**91**:799–80

201. Morrison JF, Jones PC, Meurs MF. Assessing physiological benefit from domiciliary nebulised bronchodilators in severe airflow limitation. *Eur Respir J* 1992;**5(4)**:424–9

202. Mesitz H, Copland JM, App B, McDonald CF. Comparison of outpatient nebulised vs metered dose inhaler terbutaline in chronic airflow obstruction. *Chest* 1989;**96**:1237–40

203. Jenkins SC, Heaton RW, Fulton TJ *et al.* Comparison of domiciliary nebulized salbutamol and salbutamol from a metered-dose inhaler in stable chronic airflow limitation. *Chest* 1987;**91(6)**:804–7

204. O'Driscoll BR, Kay EA, Taylor RJ *et al.* A long-term prospective assessment of home nebulizer treatment. *Respir Med* 1992;**86**:317–25

205. O'Driscoll BR. Nebulisers for chronic obstructive pulmonary disease. *Thorax* 1997;**52(Suppl 2)**:S49–S52

206. Medical Research Council Working Group. Long term domiciliary oxygen therapy in chronic hypoxic cor pulmonale complicating chronic bronchitis emphysema. *Lancet* 1981;**1**:681–6

207. Nocturnal Oxygen Therapy Trial Group. Continuous or nocturnal oxygen therapy in hypoxaemic chronic obstructive lung disease. A clinical trial. *Ann Intern Med* 1980;**93**:391–8

208. Department of Health. Domiciliary oxygen therapy service. *Drug Tariff* 10. London: HMSO, 1990

209. Crockett AJ, Cranston JM, Moss JR, Alpers JH. Domiciliary oxygen for chronic obstructive pulmonary disease. (Cochrane Review). *The Cochrane Library*, Issue 4 2002. Oxford: Update Software

210. Wedzicha JA. Mechanisms of exacerbations. *Novartis Found Symp* 2001;**234**:84–93 Discussion 93–103

211. Seemungal TAR, Donaldson GC, Paul EA *et al.* Effect of exacerbation on quality of life in patients with chronic obstructive pulmonary disease. *Am J Respir Crit Care Med* 1998;**157**:1418–22

212. Murphy TF, Sethi S, Neidermasn MS. The role of bacteria in exacerbations of COPD. A constructive view. *Chest* 2000;**118(1)**:204–9

213. Wedzicha JA, Seemungal TAR. Current thinking on the nature of exacerbation and the time course and recovery of exacerbations of COPD. In Wedzicha J, Ind P, Miles A (eds). *The Effective Management of Chronic Obstructive Pulmonary Disease*. London: Aesculapius Medical Press, 2001

214. Calverley PMA. Symptomatic Bronchodilator treatment. In: Calverley PMA, Pride NB (eds). *Chronic Obstructive Pulmonary Disease*. London: Chapman & Hall, 1994

215. Anthonisen NR, Manfreda J, Warren CPW *et al.* Antibiotic therapy in exacerbations of chronic obstructive pulmonary disease. *Ann Intern Med* 1987;**106**:196–204

216. Thompson WH, Nielson CP, Carvalho *et al.* Controlled trials of oral prednisolone in outpatients with acute COPD exacerbation. *Am J Respir Crit Care Med* 1996;**1543(2 pt1)**:407–12

217. Albert RK, Martin TR, Lewis SW. Controlled clinical trials of methylprednisolone in patients with chronic bronchitis and acute respiratory insufficiency. *Ann Intern Med* 1980;**92**:753–8

218. Gravil JH, Al-Rawas OA, Cotton MM *et al.* Home treatment of exacerbations of chronic obstructive pulmonary disease by an acute respiratory assessment service. Lancet 1998;**351(9119)**:1853–5

219. Shepphard S, Harwood D, Gray A *et al.* randomised controlled trial comparing hospital; at home care with in patient hospital care. 11. Cost minimization analysis. *BMJ* 1998;**316**:1791–6

220. Morgan M, Singh SJ. Practical Pulmonary Rehabilitation. London:Chapman & Hall, 1997

221. Lacasse Y, Wong E, Guyatt GH *et al.* Meta-analysis of respioratory rehabilitation in chronic obstructive pulmonary disease. *Lancet* 1996;**348**:1115–9

222. Griffiths TL, Burr ML, Campbell IA *et al.* Results at 1 year of outpatient multidisciplinary pulmonary rehabilitation: a randomised controlled trial. *Lancet* 2000;**355**:362–8

223. Lareau SC, Zuwallack R, Carlin B *et al.* Pulmonary rehabilitation. Official Statement of the American Thoracic Society. *AJRCCM* 1999;**159**:1666–82

224. Folgering H, Dekhujzen R, Cox N, van Herwaarden C. The rationale of pulmonary rehabilitation. *Eur Respir Rev* 1991;**1(6)**:490–7

225. Hodgkin J, Conners G, Bell W. *Pulmonary Rehabilitation — Guidleines to Success*. Philadelphia: Lippincott, 1993

226. Schols AM, Wouters EF. Nutritional abnormalities and supplementatiuon in chronic obstructive pulmonary disease. *Clin Chest Med* 2000;**21(4)**:753–62

227. Schols AM, Soeters PB, Mostert R *et al.* Physiological effects of nutritional support and anabolic steroids in patients with chronic obstructive respiratory disease. A placebo-controlled randomized trial. *Am J Respir Crit Care Med* 1995;**152**:1268–74

228. Carey IM, Strachan DP, Cook DG. Effect of changes in fresh fruit consumption on ventilatory function in healthy British adults. *Am J Respir Crit Care Med* 1998;**158**:728–33

229. Strachan D, Cox B, Erzinclioglu S, *et al*. Ventilatory function and winter fresh fruit consumption in a random sample of British adults. *Thorax* 1991,**46**:624–9

230. Watson B, Margetts P, Howarth M, *et al*. The association between diet and chronic obstructive pulmonary disease in subjects selected in general practice *Eur Respir J* 2002;**20**:313–6

231. Light RW, Merrill E.J, Depars JA et al Prevalence of depression and anxiety in patients with COPD. *Chest* 1985;**87**:35–8

232. Borak J, Sliwinski PP, Piasecki Z *et al*. Psychological status of COPD patients on long term oxygen therapy. *Eur Respir J* 1991;**4**:59–62

233. Nicholas PK, Leuner JD. Relationship between body image and chronic obstructive pulmonary disease. *Appl Nurs Res* 1992;**5**:83–8

234. Niederman MS, Clemente PH, Fein AM *et al*. Benefits of a multidisciplinary rehabilitation program. Chest 1991;**4**:798–804

235. Keele-Card G, Foxall MJ, Barron CR. Loneliness, depression, and social support of patients with COPD and their spouses. *Public Health Nurs* 1993;**10**:245–51

236. Karajgi BR, Rifkin A, Doddi S, Kelli R *et al*. The prevalence of anxiety disorders in patients with chronic obstructive pulmonary disease. *Am J Psychiatr* 1990; **147**:200–1

237. McSweeny AJ, Grant I, Heaton RK *et al* . Life quality of patients with chronic obstructive pulmonary disease. *Arch Intern Med* 1982; **142**:473–8

238. Maanen JG, Budels PJE, Dekkers FW *et al*. Risk of depression in patients with chronic obstructive pulmonary disease and its determinants. *Thorax* 2000;**57**:412-416

239. Kaplan RM, Eakin EG, Ries AL. Psychosocial issues in the rehabilitation of patients with COPD. In: *Principles and Practice of Pulmonary Rehabilitation*. Philadelphia:WB Saunders, 1993

240. ACCP/AACVPR. Pulmonary Rehabilitation Guidelines Panel Pulmonary Rehabilitation. Joint ACCP,AACVPR Evidence based guidelines. Chest 1997; **112(5)**:1363–9

241. Browne G, Roberts J, Weir R *et al*. The cost of poor adjustment to chronic illness: lessons from three studies. Health and Social Care. 1993;**2**:85–93

242. Cooke M. Evaluation of impotence. *West J Med* 1986;**145**:106–10

243. Fletcher EC, Martin RJ. Sexual dysfunction and erectile impotence in chronic obstructive pulmonary disease. *Chest* 1982;**81**:413–21

244. Thompson WL. Sexual problems in chronic respiratory disease. Postgrad Med 1986 **17**:41–52

245. Scullion JE. Sex, sexuality, and chronic respiratory disease. *Geriatr Med* 2001:48–51

246. Gregory P. Patient assessment and care planning: sexuality. *Nurs Standard* 2000;**15(9)**:38–41

247. Toma TP, Geddes DM. COPD: Is there anything new? *Airways J* 2003;**1(1)**:26–8

248. Scullion J. A surgical approach for patients with end-stage emphysema. *Br J Nursing* 1999;**8(17)**:1129–33.

249. Kerstjens HA, Grien HJ, van Der Bij W. Recent advances: Respiratory medicine. *B Med J* 2001;**323**:1349–53

250. National Council for Hospice and Specialist Palliative Care Services 1995 Specialist Palliative Care: A statement of definitions. Occasional paper 8 National Council for Hospice and Specialist Palliative Care Services

251. Jennings AL, Davies AN, Higgins JPT *et al*. A systematic review of the use of opiods in the managment of dyspnoea. *Thorax* 2000;**57**:939–44

252. Meurs MF. Opioids for dyspnoea. *Thorax* 2002;**57**:922–3

253. Johnson DC. A role for phosphodiesterase type 4 inhibitors in COPD? *Lancet* 2001;**358(9276)**:256–7

254. Poole PJ, Black PN. Oral mucolytic drugs for exacerbations of chronic obstructive pulmonary disease: systematic reviw. *BM J* 2001;**322**:1271–4

255. Bjermer L, Bisgaard H, Bousquet J et al. Montelukast and fluticasone in protecting against asthma exacerbation iin adults: one year, double blind, randomised, comparative trial. BMJ 2003;**327**:891-7

256. Sutherland ER, Allmers H, Ayas NT et al. Inhaled corticosteroids reduce the progression of airflow limitation in chronic obstructive pulmonary disease: a meta-analysis. Thorax 2003;**58**:937-41

257. Szafranski W, Cukiev A, Ramirez A et al. Efficacy and safety of budesonide/formoterol in the management of chronic obstructive pulmonary diseaes. Eur Resp J 2003;**21**:74-81

258. Calverly P, Pauwels R, Vestbo J et al. Trials of inhaled steroids and long-acting beta2 agonists group. Combined salmeterol and fluticasone in the treatment of chronic obstructive pulmonary disease: a randomised controlled trial. Lancet 2003;361:449-56

259. Neville RG, Pearson MG, Richards N et al. A cost analysis on the pattern of asthma prescribing in the UK. Eur Resp J 1999;14:605-9

260. Dworsky R, Fitzgerald GA, Oates JA et al. Effect of oral prednisone on airway inflammatory mediators in atopic asthma. Am J Repir Crit Care Med 1994;149:53-9

261. National Institute for Clinical Excellence. Chronic obstructive pulmonary disease: management of adults with chronic obstructive pulmonary disease in primary and secondary care. London: NICE (in press)

Index

Notes: Page references followed by (f) indicate figures, those followed by (cs) indicate case studies, vs. indicates a comparison.

cytokines, asthma pathophysiology, 15, 15f, 17f

D

depression
    asthma and, 102–103cs
    COPD and, 94–96, 94f, 95f
    diagnosis, 95–96
desensitization therapy, asthma prevention, 33
diazepam, 98
diet and nutrition
    asthma management, 33
    COPD exacerbations, 90–91, 91f
drug treatment see pharmacological therapy
dry powder inhalers (DPIs), 48
dyspnoea
    differential diagnoses and causes, 98, 100f
    MRC scale, 92f
    non-specific, 93
    treatment, 91–92

E

emphysema, 62, 97–98, 101cs
endotoxin exposure, asthma, 12
environmental factors, asthma, 10–11, 11f
eosinophils, asthma pathophysiology, 14–16, 15f
epidemiology
    asthma, 8, 9–10
    COPD, 8, 60–62, 61f
exacerbations see asthma exacerbations; COPD exacerbations
exercise-induced asthma, 47
exercise testing, asthma diagnosis, 19–20

F

face masks, oxygen, 85
feneterol, 107, 119
fluticasone, 34, 80, 111, 112, 118, 120
    salmeterol and, 39
forced expiratory volume in 1 second (FEV1)
    asthma, 22

COPD, 65–69, 68f
forced vital capacity (FVC)
    asthma, 22
    COPD, 65–68
formoterol, 38, 45, 78, 107, 115
    budesonide and, 39
free radicals
    asthma pathophysiology, 16
    COPD pathophysiology, 63f
functional (non-organic) disease, asthma vs., 29f

G

gastro-oesophageal reflux, asthma vs., 29f
gene–environment interactions, asthma, 11–14, 11f, 12f, 13f, 14f
General Practice Airways Group, 18
genetic factors
    alpha-antitrypsin deficiency, COPD, 64
    asthma, 10–11, 11f, 102cs
GOLD guidelines, COPD management, 78f
GPs with a special interest (GPwSIs), 58

H

Haemophilus influenzae, COPD, 81
histamine provocation tests, asthma diagnosis, 25
home treatment
    COPD exacerbations, 85
    dyspnoea, 92
hygiene hypothesis, 11–14, 12f, 13f
    allergen exposure, 12
    breastfeeding and, 12–13
    endotoxin exposure, 12
    infectious agent exposure, 13
    T-lymphocyte driven immunity, 12–13, 13f

I

immune response, asthma, 12–13, 12f, 13f
immunoglobulin E (IgE) in asthma, 15
    allergy testing, 23, 25

140